....

Fear

and

AIDS/

HIV

D0565843

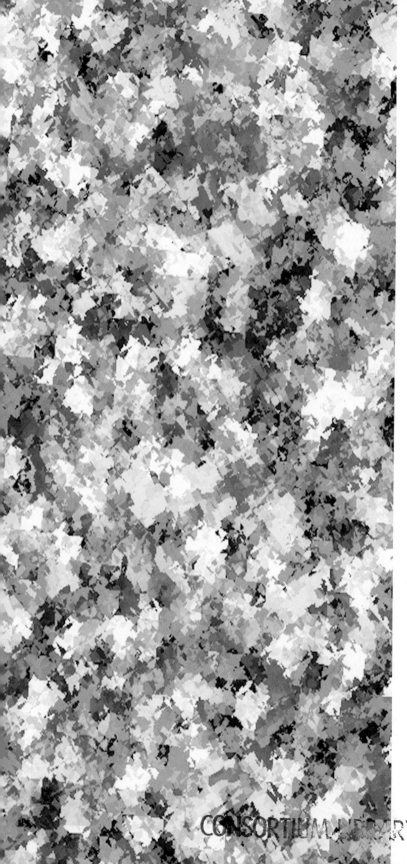

Fear and AIDS/ HIV:

Empathy and Communication

Suzanne Lego, RN, PhD, CS, FAAN

Director, Advanced Certificate Program/Psychoanalytical Training Columbia University School of Nursing

Private Practice in New York City, Pittsburgh, and Kent, Ohio

Delmar Publishers Inc.™

I（T）P™

Notice to the Reader

Publisher does not warrant or guarantee any of the products described herein or perform any independent analysis in connection with any of the product information contained herein. Publisher does not assume, and expressly disclaims, any obligation to obtain and include information other than that provided to it by the manufacturer.

The reader is expressly warned to consider and adopt all safety precautions that might be indicated by the activities described herein and to avoid all potential hazards. By following the instructions contained herein, the reader willingly assumes all risks in connection with such instructions.

The publisher makes no representations or warranties of any kind, including but not limited to, the warranties of fitness for particular purpose or merchantability, nor are any such representations implied with respect to the material set forth herein, and the publisher takes no responsibility with respect to such material. The publisher shall not be liable for any special, consequential or exemplary damages resulting, in whole or in part, from the readers' use of, or reliance upon, this material.

Cover Design: J² Designs

Delmar staff:
Publisher: David C. Gordon
Senior Acquisitions Editor: Bill Burgower
Assistant Editor: Debra M. Flis
Project Editor: Danya M. Plotsky
Production Coordinator: Barbara A. Bullock
Art and Design Coordinators: Megan K. DeSantis
   Timothy J. Conners

For information, address

Delmar Publishers Inc.
3 Columbia Circle, Box 15015
Albany, NY 12212-5015

Copyright © 1994 by Delmar Publishers Inc.

The trademark ITP is used under license.

Printed in the United States of America
Published simultaneously in Canada
by Nelson Canada,
a division of The Thomson Corporation

1   2   3   4   5   6   7   8   9   10   XXX   00   99   98   97   96   95   94

Library of Congress Cataloging-in-Publication Data

Lego, Suzanne.
   Fear and AIDS/HIV : empathy and communication / Suzanne Lego.
      p.   cm. -- (Real nursing series)
   Includes index.
   ISBN 0-8273-6155-6
   1. AIDS (Disease)—Psychosocial aspects. 2. AIDS (Disease)—Social aspects. 3. AIDS (Disease)—Nursing. 4. AIDS phobia.   I. Title II. Series.
      [DNLM: 1. Acquired Immunodeficiency Syndrome—psychology. 2. HIV Infections—psychology. 3. Fear. 4. Sociology, Medical—methods. 5. Communication. 6. Empathy. 7. Nurse-Patient Relations. WD308
   L516f   1993]
   RC607.A26L425   1993
   362.1'969792—dc20
   DNLM/DLC
   for Library of Congress   93-30743
                                                                                                        CIP

RealNursing Series
Alice M. Stein, MA, RN, Series Editor
Medical College of Pennsylvania

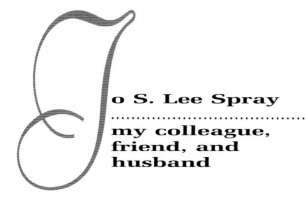

To S. Lee Spray

my colleague,
friend, and
husband

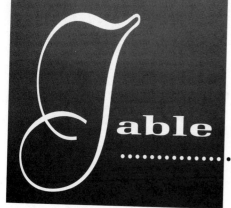
Table of Contents

APPENDIXES ■ 99

REFERENCES ■ 125

INDEX ■ 133

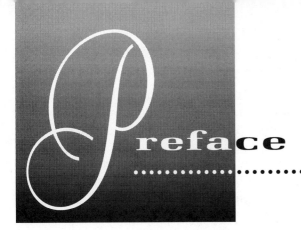

Preface

The World Health Organization estimates that 5 to 10 million people are infected with the human immunodeficiency virus (HIV). Approximately 1 million of them live in the United States. It is estimated that 1 million additional Americans are HIV positive and undiagnosed. The greatest proportion of persons with AIDS in the United States are still male homosexuals. However, the proportion of intravenous drug abusers, their wives, and their children is rapidly growing.

AIDS has been called the most serious public health issue in the world, and it is likely to become the major mental health problem of the 1990s. Psychiatric problems associated with AIDS include organic mental syndrome, dysphoria, panic disorder, major depression, substance abuse, and sleep disorders.

HIV affects not only those who have the virus but those who irrationally fear infection (AFRAIDS), those at risk who fear infection (the Worried Well), friends, families, professional and volunteer care-givers, and neighbors. Even the geriatric population has become involved, as middle-aged offspring become infected and come home to live with their parents until they die.

Every nurse in America, therefore, is likely to be faced with patients who are either in the HIV spectrum from AFRAIDS to AIDS or are involved with someone who is. We must be prepared to recognize the psychosocial effects on these people's lives and to intervene as appropriate.

To this end the book is divided into seven chapters. Chapters 1 to 3 concern the psychosocial aspects of persons in the HIV spectrum, beginning with the early stage, the middle stage, and finally the late stage. Chapter 4 addresses group therapy with HIV-infected persons. This has been found to be the most commonly employed psychological modality. Chapter 5 discusses families and friends of persons in the HIV spectrum, and Chapter 6 the professional care-givers. Chapter 7 was written by a nurse who died of AIDS in 1992. Her moving description of her experience exemplifies many of the points made throughout the book. Finally, the appendixes provide extensive lists regarding journal and newsletter publishers, helping organizations, political action groups, professional organizations, regional education and training centers, special interest groups, substance abuse publications, technical information, telephone information lines, and women's issues.

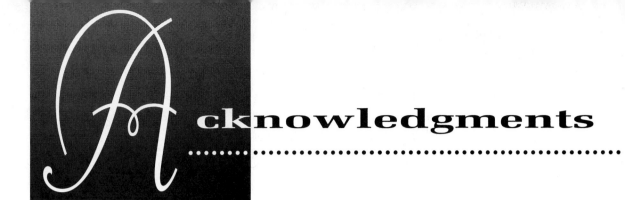

Acknowledgments

I would like to acknowledge the help of my editor, Bill Burgower, who has now seen me through two books. Thanks also to Joyce Anastasi, Ph.D., R.N., Director of the AIDS Subspeciality Program at Columbia University School of Nursing, for her expert consultation. I must also thank my expert typist, Stewart Brisby, who not only types my work but corrects and critiques it as well! Last but not least I thank my husband who is always available for sociological consultation, help, encouragement, and love.

Chapter 1

Persons in the HIV Spectrum: Early Stage

It's hard to imagine a nurse in America who has not either personally known or cared for someone who has HIV disease. To attempt to understand the psychosocial aspects of HIV disease, imagine the following scenario: You haven't been feeling well lately so you go to a doctor. After running a few tests, the doctor says, "I'm sorry to have to tell you this, but you are HIV positive." You discover that the average length of life following diagnosis is three years. You realize you will probably be dead before five years have passed. Perhaps many of your friends are dead already, or dying.

AFRAIDS

Most HIV-infected persons have had this horrifying experience. But the HIV spectrum of individuals that nurses care for also include those who have not engaged in risk behaviors but who fear getting AIDS and those who fear being diagnosed as HIV positive because they have engaged in risk behaviors. A person in the AFRAIDS group has never had unprotected sex, has never used intravenous (IV) drugs, is not a hemophiliac, and has never had a blood transfusion, but remains terrified of AIDS. In other words, individuals in the AFRAIDS group are not at serious risk, but have nonetheless become obsessed with getting the disease. People in this group would benefit from a referral for psychiatric evaluation. They will likely be treated with psychotherapy, and may be given anti-anxiety agents.

THE WORRIED WELL

A second group in the HIV spectrum is made up of those who are fearful of being diagnosed HIV positive because they *have* engaged in risk behaviors such as unprotected sex or sharing needles. For these people life can become a prolonged period of "waiting for the ax to fall," even if they are without symptoms. This group is called the *Worried Well*.

You might ask why they don't simply end the suspense by getting tested every so often, while refraining from risk behaviors. Many experts believe that taking prophylactic drugs once a person is HIV positive delays the diagnosis of AIDS, though this theory has recently come under attack. Nevertheless, the worried person might prolong life by getting tested and following a wellness-enhancing life-style.

There are several reasons why people decide not to be tested. The first is the feeling it would be "all downhill" if they tested HIV positive. Since people who test positive eventually die of AIDS, learning one is HIV positive may mean no hope of survival, at least until a cure is developed. And many believe that having some hope is better than having no hope at all.

A second reason why people don't get tested is the risk of disclosure to others. People often fear, with good reason, that once insurance companies, employers, landlords, and others learn of positive HIV status, disaster could ensue. Health insurance could be cancelled, depriving the person of necessary care. It is estimated that each person with HIV disease spends $100,000 on health care from diagnosis to death. Persons with AIDS have been known to lose jobs, apartments, friends, and even contact with family. So, some members of the Worried Well decide to "let sleeping dogs lie."

As nurses we must respect each person's decision. However, it is helpful to provide information about the benefits of being tested and the possible benefit of taking prophylactic drugs. Because these persons become panic-stricken at any potential symptom of HIV-related infections, such as coughs, night sweats, enlarged lymph nodes, or diarrhea, as nurses we want to help them get diagnosed and treated promptly for their ailments.

TESTING

Should persons decide to be tested, it is important that they know the potential social risks. Agencies that provide testing must have clear policies about the confidentiality of results. In some states, for example in New York and California, certain health professionals can inform sexual partners about positive HIV status if they believe them to be at risk and uninformed. This can be done without permission of the HIV-positive person. However, the person must be notified of this possibility *before* being tested. The nurse who is involved might encourage persons to inform partners themselves.

The Centers for Disease Control (CDC) recommends guidelines for pre- and posttest counseling. The person is told about the test and what its results can mean. Because both false negatives and false positives can occur, tests are often repeated using a different procedure, different specimens, or a different facility.

INITIAL REACTIONS TO THE DIAGNOSIS

Reactions to learning that one is HIV positive are as varied as the persons who receive the news. There are, however, common early psychological phenomena. Often people feel shock, anger, and panic. They may demonstrate denial through statements such as "There must be some mistake. This can't be true."

Shock, Anger, and Panic

Persons in high-risk groups who have dreaded hearing this news for years and who have buried many friends may have an odd first reaction of relief: at least the waiting is over. This reaction is generally short-lived and often followed by fear. Those who have lost friends are all too aware of the potential devastation of the disease in social, psychological, and physical terms.

Disappointment, Loss, and Sadness

What generally follows next is a sense of disappointment, loss, and sadness. At this early point the HIV-infected person is not really able to mobilize strength and defenses but is in need of calm, stable emotional connection with the nurse. Quiet reassurance allows the person to slowly absorb what is happening and what must or can be done.

At this point the HIV-infected person may begin to fear rejection and abandonment. Close, accepting family and friends can help reassure the person that they will stick by them. But unfortunately, in the highest risk groups, families often view the infected persons as having brought the disease on themselves, and reject or abandon them outright. The nurse who is in contact with family and friends can be very helpful in encouraging them not to abandon their loved ones and in helping them find support from others. In the case of persons who are relatively alone, the nurse can help them find support groups and agencies to help them through this period.

Fear

HIV-infected persons may at this point begin to fear incapacitation, physical and mental deterioration, deformity, and pain, especially if they have witnessed the illness and death of friends. A person I counseled had been at the bedside of his brother when he died a terrible death, vomiting and hemorrhaging at the end. The nurse can help by allowing the person to say anything, no matter how horrifying, and listening in a calm, emotionally connected way. This talk helps the person to become relatively desensitized and is far better than denial and dissociation. The nurse can even reassure the person that there will be professionals there to help.

Shame

A sense of shame, self-blame, and fear of stigma often occurs. The knowledge that one has a terminal disease is always devastating. But when the disease is viewed by others as a "punishment" for "bad" behavior, the results are doubly devastating. Under these circumstances it is very hard for the person to feel whole and good. In many cases, the person's own behavior is in no way connected to contracting the disease, for example, in cases of hemophilia, children who are infected by mothers through the bloodstream, or those who were infected by a blood transfusion. However, because the disease carries such social stigma, the person suffers the phenomenon of "blaming the victim."

In the case of the person who contracted the virus through sexual contact or sharing needles, the blame and shame may come from both internal and external sources. The gay or bisexual man may feel guilty about his sexuality, the woman about her relationships with bisexuals or drug abusers, and drug users about their status in life. Women often have the added burden of guilt regarding their children's futures. Nurses must examine their own feelings about this shame and blame. If a nurse believes that HIV-infected persons have brought the disease on themselves, that nurse, through discussion with a supervisor, should examine how this negative thinking affects both the nurse and HIV-infected person.

A person I counseled entered therapy because he wanted to understand his bisexuality from an interpersonal standpoint. He said, "I can face death, but I want to understand how this all happened, and to resolve my guilt about what I have done to my family." Through several years of insight-oriented psychodynamic therapy he was able to accomplish this. In the majority of cases, therapy is conducted in groups and is supportive rather than insight-oriented.

Denial

Another reaction to an HIV diagnosis is denial. We have all heard of people who ignore the diagnosis through the process of dissociation and then go on having unsafe sex. A person might think, "I can lick this," or might refuse to think of it at all. Such denial can have serious consequences: the HIV-infected person is not likely to benefit from the health care that *is* available for lengthening and improving life, and risks infecting sexual partners. Nurses can be of assistance by gently helping the person to accept the HIV–positive status.

Suicidal Thoughts

Suicidal thoughts may occur after the person has accepted the diagnosis. These thoughts may be fleeting, for example, "Maybe I should end it all now and get it over with," or an actual plan may be instituted. The HIV-positive person may want to protect family and friends from the pain of the prolonged illness and death, or may fear dementia or a painful death.

When suicide is mentioned the nurse must assess the risk by determining (1) whether the person means to carry out a plan very soon or is thinking about doing so in the future, (2) whether something besides the diagnosis has just occurred, (3) if the person has a well-thought-out plan, (4) if the person has immediate available means of committing suicide, and (5) if there is a support system available. Often the mention of suicide is a cry for help and psychotherapy should be instituted at once. If there *is* clear danger, the nurse has an obligation to act at once to avert the suicide. The issue of "rational suicide" will be discussed in Chapter 2.

The Ego Chill

Reality of certain death and what Erik Erikson called "the ego chill" may also occur. Erikson (1958) described the ego chill as "A shudder that comes from sudden awareness that our non-existence . . . is entirely possible." The nurse is often in a position to help the person explore feelings about death. In fact, in many cases the person may have no one else to talk to about this. Often family and friends eschew such discussions, saying, "They may find a cure before then," or "That's a long way off," or "Just think positively." A person I counseled talked at length about never seeing his children grow up, as well as seeing his dead relatives in heaven after death. He often said, "You're the only person I can discuss this with."

ADDRESSING THE PSYCHOSOCIAL NEEDS IN THE EARLY STAGE

Persons who are newly diagnosed as HIV positive will receive posttest counseling at the testing facility. Following this a number of options are possible. The person may decide to enter individual counseling with a professional therapist, in some cases a master's or doctorally prepared nurse. The nurse who enters into a therapy relationship with the HIV-infected person should do so with a strong sense of commitment, realizing this will probably involve helping the person through a number of illnesses to death. The nurse may receive many panicky phone calls, make hospital and home visits, watch the person deteriorate physically, and perhaps be present at death. Obviously, this kind of therapy is not entered into lightly. The nurse must be able to discuss death and dying in a relatively comfortable way. I was counseling a client who was able to discuss his impending death with me. I thought I was comfortable with our discussions, until my unconscious gave me away. One day we spent most of the session discussing his impending death. At the end of the session, as I walked him to the door, he suddenly asked, "What time is it?" We discovered that I was attempting to end his session 15 minutes early! He came back into the office and we resumed the session. He asked, "Do you think you dismissed me early because we were talking about my death?" I replied, "I thought I was used to the idea, but I guess I'm still anxious about it." He then asked, "How can we *ever* get used to it?"

By far the most common form of counseling for newly diagnosed persons is the support group. Even before AIDS, we learned that support groups for persons with terminal illness, for example cancer patients, are helpful both in promoting psychological well-being and prolonging life. There is a great deal of evidence that social support increases both mental and physical well-being regardless of the person's illness. The nurse can be helpful in referring the person to a support group. The value of these groups will be further explored in Chapter 4.

Education about HIV is very important at the time of diagnosis. The HIV-infected person wants primarily to know the prognosis, treatment, and answers to questions about life-style. Flaskerud (1992, p. 248) suggests that specific areas for education include

- **Reconfirmation of test results on a second serum specimen in a reference laboratory**
- **Interpretation of the results (includes the information that the person does not have AIDS)**
- **Evaluation for suicide potential**
- **Crisis intervention counseling as needed**
- **Information on whom to tell: partners, health care providers, blood and organ donation centers**
- **Information on alternative test sites for partners**
- **Discussion of follow-up for partners and children**
- **Referral to a partner notification program, if needed**
- **Information on transmission, safer sex and drug use practices, and reinfection**
- **Information on pregnancy and perinatal transmission**
- **Information on symptoms associated with the spectrum of HIV disease**
- **Referral to an early intervention program that includes attention to life-style practices that may suppress the immune system and activate the disease**

- Referral to an HIV-positive persons' support group
- Referral for medical follow-up
- Referral for drug rehabilitation program
- Information on entering experimental protocols
- Referral for psychologic, social, and psychiatric services, as needed
- Discussion of potential discrimination and effects on housing, employment, insurance, and so forth

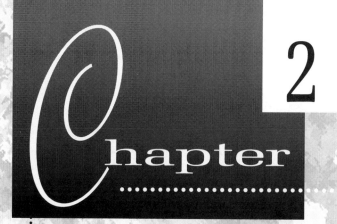

Chapter 2

Persons in the HIV Spectrum: Middle Stage

REACTIONS TO THE ILLNESS

Loss of Control

The person who has moved from relatively healthy HIV–positive status to an opportunistic infection might consider this the beginning of the end. But it in fact may not be. For example, the person may develop Kaposi's sarcoma early on, yet remain in relatively good health and go on to live several more years without other symptoms. Yet nonetheless, one of the first reactions to the onset of an infection is the feeling of having lost control of one's life.

It is natural for a person to feel out of control as the virus progresses. The nurse can help by talking with the person about what can be done to regain control. For example, some opportunistic infections can respond to long-term suppressive therapy. The nurse can best help the person by suggesting ways to stay in good physical condition, which in turn improves mental status, as the person comes to see ways to take control of life.

Helplessness and Vulnerability

Often the HIV-infected person feels both vulnerable and helpless. In fact, the term "opportunistic infection" suggests that infections are out there just waiting to strike. This way of thinking only increases stress, and we know that stress is detrimental to the immune system.

But at this stage, the person is not helpless. The nurse can point out the benefits of healthy living, good diet, exercise, meditation, and relaxation. HIV-infected persons can also be encouraged to reach out to others for assistance, and more importantly, become involved in helping others. Helping others can add meaning to daily life, as well as help the person leave something of value behind. Often HIV-infected people become in-volved politically, for example, in AIDS activism; devote their creative endeavors to the arts, by writing about their experiences in plays, novels, or journals; or become active on a local level in AIDS social agencies, such as the Gay Men's Health Crisis in New York City, the Shanti Project in San Francisco, and so forth. All of these activities affirm that the person is not helpless against the disease.

Feeling of Passivity and Victimization

Along with vulnerability comes the feeling that one is passive and being victimized. Such negative thinking is, again, not conducive to health and well-being. For this reason experts and activists in the field have discouraged the use of the term "AIDS victim" and the phrase "dying of AIDS." These have been replaced with the phrases "HIV-infected person" and "living with HIV." The general idea is to view this as a chronic, life-threatening illness, as opposed to a death sentence.

Death seems to come earlier for persons who give up, who have little social support and believe they have few reasons to live. The CDC considers long-term survivors to be those who are still alive three years after AIDS diagnosis. This is somewhat ambiguous, since the criteria for diagnosis of AIDS is revised from time to time using different measures related to opportunistic infections or T-cell count. At any rate, in January 1993, *Parade* magazine interviewed a number of people who had survived at least nine years since the onset of AIDS-related symptoms.

Those interviewed all had certain characteristics in common. These included "pluck and courage to face up to almost anything, spirituality, irreverence including the ability to laugh at themselves, and a feeling they had been chosen to help others" (p. 5).

An in-depth nurses' study of three men with AIDS who were doing well identified five factors that seemed to contribute to their well-being: autonomy and mastery of their illness and life; spiritual or existential beliefs; self-acceptance; staying active and involved; and positive thinking (Kendall et al, 1989).

Severe Reduction in Self-Esteem

Chronic illness often causes people to feel less important. One reason is that illness may restrict them from the strongest sources of self-esteem in our society: love and work. Illness can drastically alter a loving relationship, producing strains and burdens on the caregiver and feelings of guilt and shame for both the ill person and caregiver. If the person is unable to work, especially if the work is very important and meaningful, self-esteem may plummet. Paul Monette, in his moving book *Borrowed Time* (1988), describes the poignant moment when his lover who has AIDS must close his law office because he is too sick to work. They arrive at the office to find everything packed up and the pictures removed from the wall. His lover dissolves into tears in a rare moment of self-pity and cries, "Oh, God."

Not only the process of work, but the work itself can be lost when the person dies. For example, artists and writers sometimes die alone, estranged from families, and with no friends alive to act as curators of their work. For this reason a project has been instituted in New York to collect and store their art after the death of persons with AIDS.

The nurse can help by talking about relationships and work, and exploring the continuing importance of existing relationships and of work left to be done, even if it must be done at home or on a different scale. One gay man with AIDS vowed to spend as much time as possible with his niece following diagnosis. Over a period of years, he took her to concerts and museums, teaching her all he could about art. This not only gave his life meaning, but helped him feel he had left something of value behind.

Self-esteem is further reduced when one has a highly stigmatized illness such as AIDS and belongs to stigmatized groups such as IV drug abusers and homosexuals. Though efforts have been made to educate the public about the transmission of HIV, most people demonstrate irrational behavior despite education and information. For example, a kind, compassionate, and intelligent doctor-friend told me a few years ago he wears a gown and mask when treating HIV-infected persons urologically. When I asked if he realized HIV was contracted through the exchange of body fluids he answered, "I don't take any chances. I have a family." Many HIV-infected persons have horror stories about this kind of treatment by health care professionals, which increases any low self-esteem the person brings to the situation.

As nurses we must be very careful to examine our own thoughts, feelings, and actions relating to HIV-infected persons. This is done within the context of our responsibility to patients. The American Nurses Association Task Force to Develop Guidelines for the Care of People with AIDS (1988) clearly states that we have a moral obligation to care for AIDS patients except in the rare instances when the nurse would clearly incur harm, for example, if the nurse is immuno-suppressed or not supplied with adequate equipment or policies to avoid risk. This care must be delivered in such a way that the dignity and self-esteem of the HIV-infected person is maintained.

Changes in Physical Appearance

Changes in physical appearance nearly always occur in HIV-infected persons. The most common is the progressive wasting away of body fat and muscle, leading to a stooped appearance as well as the striking purple marks related to Kaposi's sarcoma. These changes are difficult for most people to bear, especially those who have always taken pride in their appearance.

One of the phenomena described by HIV-infected persons, however, is a reordering of priorities. Those who are able to engage in meaningful interpersonal relations and work find that these take on more importance, while relatively superficial indices of importance such as body image or physical appearance fall away. In a moving scene from the play *Shadowboxes*, some friends have gathered to visit a dying young man. They open some champagne and it sprays someone's sport jacket. Much fuss is made over how this was allowed to happen, and who was to blame. Suddenly the dying young man shouts, "For Christ sake, it's only a jacket!," bringing everyone back to the reality of the moment.

The nurse can play a part in helping HIV-infected persons to reorder priorities and to explore what is really important to them. For many, these priorities will turn out to be their families, friends, children, and work. One person I counseled decided to concentrate on improving his relationships with his two children before he died. However, as his therapy progressed he saw that this was easier said than done. Because he was so narcissistic, he was unable to change his behavior to accomplish this task. For example, his 14-year-old son loved sports. When I suggested he watch the games on TV with his son he replied, "But I *hate* sports." We then explored his inability to put aside what *he* wanted for the good of the relationship, even temporarily. He talked about his own narcissistic parents and in time was able to change. I bring up this example to show that many of the issues raised in therapy have unconscious roots, and patience is needed to help people change. As experienced, objective nurses, it often seems obvious to us what must be done and how to do it. This is often less obvious to the infected person. The knowledge that one is dying does not necessarily change lifelong personality traits.

Sense of Isolation

Persons who are dying often experience a sense of isolation. We've all heard the old adage "we all die alone," meaning that no one, no matter how close to us, can experience our death as we do. Unfortunately, HIV-infected persons sometimes do literally die alone, estranged from family and abandoned by friends. It is for this reason the nurse, particularly the nurse psychotherapist, has such an important role to play. Nurses may be present both physically and psychologically as these persons approach their death, and may be instrumental in helping them plan who they want with them at the time of death. If the HIV-infected person can become a part of a support group, the sense of isolation can be lessened. Not all are interested in doing this. A client of mine who was married and bisexual felt no connection to gay men or to IV drug abusers and refused to investigate other possible support groups. He preferred to be with family and friends during his illness. Another said he was only "brought down" by the AIDS support group he attended. He was relatively healthy and active. "Seeing all those people sick and dying just depressed me."

As with all the psychological phenomena of people living with AIDS, each phenomenon will be experienced a little differently according to each unique personality. The wise nurse will be attuned to the special needs of each individual.

Stigma also produces separation and social isolation. Sociologists who study stigma report that the isolation may result from avoidance of others as well as from an internal, self-imposed state. Persons with leprosy who had no visible sign of the disease to the outside world sometimes lived in leprosariums, refusing to leave the grounds. It seemed they had internalized the stigma of others and chose to isolate themselves. The same phenomenon can occur with HIV-positive persons.

Guilt over Life-Style

Gay and bisexual men, IV drug abusers, and people who contracted the disease through sexual contact often feel a sense of guilt. This is frequently reinforced by family members and society at large, who may believe they "brought this on themselves." During the middle phase of the illness, there is usually time to explore feelings of guilt. In prolonged psychotherapy, for example, the person may want to discuss the roots of his homosexuality.

Homosexuality: Prevailing ideas about the cause of homosexuality have changed over time. For the first half of this century it was believed by most that family dynamics came to play in creating male homosexuality. The classic dynamic is believed to involve a smothering, close-binding mother and a distant father. Empirical evidence bears this out in many cases.

In the 1960s and 1970s this theory, and the research methods used to substantiate it, came under serious dispute. With the sexual revolution, gay men began to declare that their homosexuality was a "life choice" not dictated by family background. During this period, political activism led to the Gay Rights Movement and problems of discrimination against gays were addressed. At the same time, gay rights groups were instrumental in having the term "homosexuality" removed from the Diagnostic Statistical Manual of Mental Disorders and having it replaced by "ego-dystonic homosexuality." Their belief was that homosexuality was not an illness but in many cases an ego-syntonic choice.

With the onset of the AIDS epidemic in the 1980s, the concept of the gay life-style as a free choice became problematic. Homophobics and members of the conservative far-right in America could then use this reasoning against gay men with AIDS, saying, "You brought this on yourself by 'choosing' to be gay."

In addition, while it has always been hard for many gay men to accept the family dynamics theory, when the family was needed for care it became even harder to accept this theory on an unconscious and sometimes even conscious level. Besides this, another political movement spearheaded by the National Alliance for Mental Illness (NAMI) was utterly opposed to the theory of family dynamics, for they saw this as "blaming" the mother or father.

In the 1980s studies began to appear in professional journals and in lay magazines and newspapers linking homosexuality to genetic, hormonal, or biochemical etiology. In the 1990s, called the Decade of the Brain, a great deal of behavior is attributed to biochemical causes. This explanation has found fertile ground in the gay community; it frees both the family and the gay person of any responsibility for the homosexuality. However, no conclusive evidence has been found to support a biological theory of etiology.

Whatever the cause of homosexuality, gay men often believe it is their homosexuality that is to blame for contracting HIV. The nurse can be helpful in hearing the person out, helping him explore his tangled feelings of guilt, blame, or shame, and helping him to see that no one and nothing is to blame. The goal is to achieve an existential point of view. "This has all happened. This is my experience now. What can I do to make the most of the time I have left?"

IV Drug Abuse: For the IV drug abuser, the picture is somewhat similar. Many come from urban slums and grew up in neighborhoods where everyone they knew used drugs, including their caregivers. Studies of persons abusing drugs have found that nearly all have one or more psychiatric disorders that have existed over a lifetime. These include generalized anxiety disorder, antisocial personality disorder, phobias, psychosexual dysfunction, major depression, and dysthymia. Owing to the profound deprivation of care and support in early development, many lifetime drug users have the primitive, impulsive personalities characteristic of addictive personality disorder. Who is responsible for all this? Many would say the societies that allow poverty to breed urban ghettos. Others would say the families, and still others that these individuals have "brought this on themselves." Some even go so far as to say society would be improved by the deaths of all these people, whom they see as symbols of crime, disease, and the degeneration of society. In light of these attitudes, it is easy to see why IV drug abusers feel guilty, bewildered, and apathetic. Often poor or in prisons, they believe they have little to be proud of in life.

Nurses can play a very important role in helping these persons resolve their guilt and move to a more existential viewpoint. Spirituality and religion can be helpful when forgiveness can be tied to God or to spirituality in whatever form the person chooses.

Individual families, as well as certain sectors of society, may believe that illness and death are retribution for HIV-infected persons' sexual behavior. In prisons and hospitals HIV-infected persons are often feared and mistreated by personnel.

The nurse can be helpful by providing a close, professional, interpersonal relationship with the person. By treating the person with respect and dignity, promoting honest communication, and encouraging relationships with others in the same situation, this connection of illness and retribution can begin to unravel. Chaplains, priests, ministers, and rabbis who are free of this irrational connection can also provide help and support.

Anger and Acting Out

It is hard to imagine having a terminal disease and not feeling angry. HIV-infected persons react with anger and act out on a continuum. At one extreme is the person who says "I got this thing, I'm gonna die, and I'm taking as many people with me as possible!" This is a relatively rare reaction. Toward the middle of the continuum is the person who from time to time becomes angry or even enraged at the life that is being stolen or at the insensitivity of health care providers. This anger is to be expected. In Larry Kramer's moving play *The Destiny of Me*, about an AIDS activist hospitalized with AIDS, there is a dramatic moment when the patient throws plastic bags of "blood" all over the room, splattering the walls. In that moment the audience experiences the rage as well as its futility. At the other extreme is the person who buries the anger and becomes depressed and apathetic.

In each case the nurse has an important role to play. For the angry person who acts out and endangers the lives of others, psychotherapy is indicated immediately. If the nurse is seeing the person in psychotherapy, the goal is to help the person express the anger and rage in the session so that aggression outside the office is decreased. The nurse helps the person explore all the possible elements of the rage, for example the losses, the injustice, the betrayal, the poor treatment by others, and so forth. It is only through in-depth counseling with an emotionally present second person that this anger can abate. If the acting out continues, it is likely to lead to more problems, including unconscious guilt and even violence.

When the person expresses "normal" anger, the nurse should remain empathetic and validating. "You sure have good reason to be mad." It is important to speak in plain language, avoiding what might sound like condescension or professional jargon, such as, "It will help you to express your anger in an appropriate manner." With a patient I counseled, I often shook my head sympathetically, saying "Yeah, it's enough to drive you crazy!" when he complained about the health care system. When a person is unable to get angry, depression often results. To avoid this, the nurse must help the person feel free to express anger openly.

Anger at nurses, doctors, other health care workers, the government, the Federal Drug Administration, and any others involved in the health care system is a very common phenomenon among HIV-infected persons. As with paranoia (see below), part of this feeling comes from other sources and is displaced onto the health care system, and part is reality based. Because HIV-infected persons are angry at the losses they experience, the nurse is often the unfair target of anger. Patience and understanding are required when this occurs. At the same time, we know that many abuses occur in the delivery of health care to these persons. Studies have shown that many nurses and other health care workers prefer to care for patients who do not have HIV-related disease and are biased against persons who do carry this diagnosis. While this may come from ignorance about how HIV is spread, it also results from homophobia, prejudice against IV drug abusers, and an irrational fear of being contaminated by associating with these "undesirable" people.

When complaints about the health care system occur, nurses can help patients sort out for themselves what anger is displaced and what is realistic, and encourage them to express feelings openly. As the AIDS epidemic progresses, it is hoped that a combination of education, understanding of emotional and social aspects, and governmental health care reform will alleviate some of the justifiable anger at the health care system.

Depression

Depression is very common in HIV-infected persons. There are often "peaks and valleys," and the depression occurs with the valley of bad news about the progression of the illness, for example, a drop in T-cell count, the early signs of an opportunistic infection, or a dramatic loss such as blindness from cytomegalovirus. A patient I counseled went into a profound depression following a big retirement party, a move to a smaller home, and a return from a visit to Europe where he had managed to forget he had AIDS. Upon his return the reality came crashing down on him. He became psychotic, was hospitalized, recovered, and came home only to lapse into a deep depression. He was treated with an antidepressant and his psychotherapy sessions were increased to twice a week. In a matter of two months the depression lifted. In therapy we concentrated a great deal on his anger, attempting to bring it into conscious awareness. He had spent his life trying to be a good son to his mother, but secretly acting out sexually. Though a married father, he participated in back room sex, managing to conceal this from everyone. As his therapy progressed he was able to express deep-seated rage at his early restrictive upbringing, his illness, and his impending loss of life.

Paranoia

Persons with AIDS often experience paranoia, both for unconscious reasons and for reality-based social reasons. The psychodynamics of paranoia have to do with the projection of one's own anger onto an external source. This external source is then perceived as dangerous. Full-blown paranoia can result from neurological changes or from current life circumstances. It is not uncommon for persons to develop the paranoid idea that others are out to get them. When a priest I counseled became hospitalized for psychosis, he believed his congregation all knew he was bisexual and had AIDS, though in fact they did not. In this case his own anger was projected onto others and he came to believe they were all against him. Paranoia can often be fed by reality—perhaps family members, neighbors, and co-workers *are* in fact hostile and are plotting against the person with AIDS.

Once again, the nurse can be helpful by engaging in an interpersonal relationship that is open, honest, and straightforward. In this relationship the nurse can help the person sort out what part of the paranoia is an internal projection and what part is justified. When the person I counseled was hospitalized on a psychiatric unit, I visited him there. The nurses on the unit were sensitive to his need for contact with me, the therapist who had an ongoing relationship with him. They invited me to present his case at grand rounds and later reported that it was helpful to learn about his background and psychodynamics. This information helped them to understand many of the odd behaviors he had exhibited on the unit, including delusions and hallucinations. Once he left the hospital, he and I were able to discuss both the delusions and the hallucinations in great detail, just as one would discuss the meaning of dreams. All three phenomena—dreams, delusions, and hallucinations—represent windows into the unconscious and can be understood in light of the person's current experience. For example, when I visited this patient in the hospital, I quickly determined that, although he was glad I came, he did not want me to stay long. This was evident in the polite, formal way he behaved. It was clear he had to work hard to hold himself together and he did not want me to know about his delusions and hallucinations just yet. He later confessed that one of his delusions was that he could make people disappear from life by looking at them. He was afraid to look at me for fear his power would annihilate me. We were later able to explore this as representative of his ambivalence about people in general, his anger at authority, and his overall feeling of powerlessness.

Fear of Violence

The National Association of People Living with AIDS conducted a study in 1992 in which more than 1,800 HIV-infected persons were asked their foremost concerns. The most startling finding was that fear of violence against them ranked highest. Also named were concern with poor access to health care, discrimination by health care workers, and lack of financial resources, particularly benefits and entitlements. A high number of respondents had been victims of violence. Over 21% reported that they had experienced violence outside the home, and 12% said they had been victims of domestic violence.

The nurse who learns of violent behavior against an HIV-infected person can act as an advocate for that person. This may mean exploring ways to avoid further violence or referring family members to support groups. If patients are bedridden, they may have no one else to discuss the problem with; this makes it even more important for the nurse to be attentive and empathic. Many AIDS resource centers, such as the Gay Men's Health Crisis in New York, have ombudsmen departments for reporting violence, discrimination, or unfair treatment.

Sense of Betrayal

HIV-infected persons may experience betrayal from a number of sources. First, they may be betrayed by the person who passed on the disease: a partner who was aware of being HIV positive and yet said nothing, or a partner who contracted the disease by being unfaithful. Second, partners or family members may desert the person after learning of the HIV status, which can be a cruel blow. HIV-infected persons may be betrayed by friends and associates who shun them, and health care workers who discriminate against and mistreat them. And finally, if they are religious, they may believe God has betrayed them.

When betrayal occurs, there is loss of a belief in relationships with others that was previously comforting to the person. The person can be helped by the nurse to mourn the loss of this idea or belief as it relates to a specific person or group. At the same time the nurse helps the person acquire new sources of comfort to replace the lost ones. These include the professional relationship with the nurse; new relationships, for example, in a support group; a sense of the self as a source of comfort; and if the person is spiritual, the idea of a higher being or power who can be a source of comfort and peace.

Escape into Drugs

It is not unusual for HIV-infected persons, especially IV drug abusers, to use drugs to escape the emotional and physical pain associated with AIDS. This is obviously disconcerting if the person is sharing needles with unsuspecting partners.

Nurses are often stymied by how to confront this problem. While there is no easy answer, a close, ongoing relationship with the person may be of some help, as may a support group. Inner-city support groups for HIV-infected persons have been found helpful in dealing with this problem of drug abuse among members.

In cases of street drugs used to control pain, the nurse can help the person obtain health care including evaluation for medication.

Somatic Preoccupation

As might be expected, HIV-infected persons become extremely preoccupied with bodily functions and potential symptoms of opportunistic infections. T-cell counts may become a constant preoccupation. There is a sense of constantly waiting for the sword to drop.

The nurse is in a position to offer education, support, and encouragement. Attention must be paid to staying well between illnesses, with an emphasis on a healthy diet, exercise, meditation, and relaxation—which is especially important, since stress reduces the immune system's ability to function. Our work with HIV-infected persons should exemplify Florence Nightingale's belief: that the nurse's role is to keep the patient in the best possible state for the body's natural abilities to take over and heal.

Projective Identification

This phenomenon occurs when persons take unwanted aspects of themselves and unconsciously place them in another. This leads to a feeling of relief from the unwanted emotion. Melanie Klein first described this when she spoke of babies infusing their mothers with unwanted aggression and then remaining identified with the mothers through this infusion. Psychiatric nurses observe this phenomenon with borderline personality patients who infuse them with anger, aggression, pity, and so forth. This same phenomenon has been observed in persons with HIV disease. Because there are so many very frightening, unwanted feelings, there is often an attempt to remove them and place them in others.

For this to occur, the nurse or another party must unconsciously participate through the process of *introjective identification*; that is, the nurse must be unconsciously willing to accept the projection. For example, the person might shout, "What *good* are you to me? I'm going to die anyway." The nurse may suddenly feel the same anger and helplessness the person is expressing. The alert and sensitive nurse will be aware of this process when it happens and attempt to step back from the situation. It is helpful to the person if the nurse can receive the message with empathy and avoid being caught up in the person's panic.

SPECIAL CONCERNS

Questions about Whether and How to Tell Loved Ones

We live in an age when many believe that everyone should know everything about everybody else, hence the plethora of tell-all talk shows. As someone observed recently, "Never before have so *many* known so *much* about people they care so little about." For HIV-infected persons, the question about whether and when to tell loved ones is a serious and sometimes controversial one. There is little doubt that telling current sex partners one is HIV positive is the right thing to do. However, it is not an easy thing to do. The nurse might therefore be called upon to help the person with this task, either by counseling the person before or after the encounter or being present during it. It is best if the person is prepared for any response, for the encounter might be very dramatic and is likely to be very upsetting to all involved. If the person is in therapy with the nurse, an appointment could be scheduled just after the event for that person alone or with the partner. Testing of the partner usually follows, as well as the pretest and posttest counseling.

Telling elderly parents is another consideration. Today it is fairly unusual to withhold this information, but in cases where family members are very old and in precarious health themselves, HIV-infected persons may wish to spare them this blow.

Telling children is especially painful. Many parents decide against this for a number of reasons. The first is the fear that it will adversely affect the child because of the period of development the child or teenager is passing through. A bisexual person and his wife decided not to tell their 14-year-old son as he was just entering adolescence and going through the normal identity crises of that period. Neither did they tell their daughter, a senior in high school who was busily planning to go off to college. Wrapped up in school activities, her prom, and graduation, she would certainly have been traumatized by this news. The couple reasoned it would be better to tell their children later, when they were in different life phases. Little children can be severely traumatized, since their understanding of death is incomplete. They are left to worry constantly about whether the parent is getting sick and going to die. Another reason to withhold this information has to do with stigma and discrimination. Children cannot be expected to withhold such upsetting information from others, and once it is disclosed they may become the victims of discrimination, further complicating their lives.

However, it becomes very difficult to maintain such a secret. Frequent doctor visits, lots of medicines to take, and whispered conferences between parents alert the child that something is wrong. In the case of the person with teenaged children, the parents decided to tell a half-truth. The father did develop lymphoma, so the children and friends of the family were told he had cancer. This seemed a logical explanation for his weakness and loss of weight. When he was admitted to the hospital, considerable pressure was brought to bear on both he and his wife to tell the children. As their psychotherapist, I was asked by them to explain to hospital personnel why this secret was being kept. Interestingly, the nurses understood and readily accepted the family's choice. Other team members did not, and one psychiatrist began to call me repeatedly, urging me to encourage the parents to disclose this "family secret." Finally the parents had to ask that he not call or contact them or me again. This is an interesting example of health care professionals insisting they know what's best for families rather than letting the family decide for themselves what *they* want.

There are, to be sure, some benefits to disclosure. Children may be better able to cope with the stress of illness if they can talk openly and honestly with their parents. The sense of isolation they may feel is lessened if they are not shut out of the parent's secret.

Nurses can be helpful in talking with clients about how and when to tell children, listening carefully to the parent's motivation to tell or not tell. One father wanted to tell his children because they would be more likely, he believed, to do as he said if they knew he was dying. I pointed out that this was the equivalent of emotional blackmail! A small book entitled *How*

Can I Tell You? was published by the Association for the Care of Children's Health and is helpful in dealing with this issue. (For a list of children's books on death, dying, and AIDS see the reference section of this book.)

Questions about Intimacy and Sexuality after Diagnosis

While loss of interest in sex is common in the period following diagnosis, as the person begins to feel better, libido often returns. While we all know that the only safe sex is abstinence, "safer sex" can be practiced by those who are HIV positive, through mutual masturbation, touching, and hugging. (While condom use reduces risk, it is not 100% safe, and psychological and social factors may prevent condom use.) For many, sex is a way to obtain the nongenital contact for which all human beings yearn, that is, hugging, stroking, cuddling, and other forms of closeness. HIV-infected persons who are abstinent sometimes report that this is one of the hardest things about being HIV positive. As one man said, "I long for physical closeness, the warmth and comfort of a body next to mine."

The nurse can be helpful in providing information about safer sex and in exploring the person's experience with both sex and intimacy. One person I counseled was engaged in an affair with a man who knew my client was HIV positive. As time went on and my client became weaker, his partner began to withdraw sexually. I pointed out this probably was a result of his lover's anticipatory grief: he was increasingly afraid to enjoy their sex and intimacy as the time to part grew closer. I encouraged him to talk this over with his lover and to tell him what he himself was experiencing.

Reconciliation with Estranged Family Members

Because of the stigma associated with AIDS, homosexuality, and IV drug abuse, HIV-infected persons are often estranged from their families. As the illness progresses, there is often a desire for reconciliation on the part of the infected person. It is not easy to die alone, and even if the person has friends, a lover, or a nuclear family, there is often the desire to leave the world on good terms with one's parents. This in fact may symbolize the ultimate "forgiveness" for the guilt or shame felt about one's life-style or contracting AIDS.

The nurse can help the person explore feelings about estranged family members. Though the person may profess no interest whatsoever in reconciliation, this tough, extreme stance may cover a longing for acceptance and a fear of rejection. The person can be gently helped to explore all the feelings about family members, both positive and negative, and to examine why attempts at reconciliation could or could not occur. Of course, the nurse should have no vested interest in convincing the person either way. If nurses begin to feel strongly in either direction, a talk with another professional is advised. The person may also want the nurse present for support or may need to talk just after the reconciliation experience.

The "Limbo" Phase

Once the initial responses to diagnosis have died down, treatment has begun, and opportunistic infections are in check, persons begin to feel better, sometimes even healthy. At this point they may say, "I think I'm going to beat this. I can almost forget I have AIDS," or, as one of my clients said, "I've been gearing up to die, what am I going to do if I live?" Because we know that HIV disease eventually results in death, we can assume that two phenomena are operating here. One is a brief psychological respite fed by denial. The other is an unconscious continuing awareness that all is not really well. HIV-infected persons have described this as a bittersweet period: "If only it could stay like this."

The nurse is aware that the valley following this peak is often a low one. Because the person has felt so relatively healthy, it is very distressing to become sick again. The nurse encourages an "enjoy-the-moment" philosophy but is alert for depression following the elation.

Unfinished Business

As the disease progresses, the need to complete unfinished business and to get one's affairs in order increases. This may involve unresolved personal relationships, legal matters, and even plans for the funeral or memorial service. A person I counseled said his loved ones were encouraging him to do just that, but he could not bring himself to because it seemed to indicate the beginning of the end and meant "giving in." I gently pointed out that getting one's affairs in order and "the beginning of the end" have nothing to do with each other: that making plans would not hasten his funeral. Others want to plan everything, for it provides some sense of control. Still others say, "I'll get things in order, but I have no intention of dying any time soon!" As with each phenomenon, the nurse moves along at the person's own pace, offering support and the opportunity to talk and express emotion openly.

Resurrection Fantasies as Others Recover from an Infection

In support groups for HIV-infected persons, there is occasional coming and going as people are hospitalized, recover, and return. When they do not return, there is despair. When they do, the phenomenon of resurrection fantasy may occur.

As with other forms of temporary denial, nurses help the person to talk about thoughts, feelings, wishes, and dreams. Nurses are careful to be realistic but not negativistic. For example, "It's good to see John back again. I guess we all wish it could last forever." This message carries both the positive feelings and the reality.

Resistance to Talking about Death

It has been said that "no one can look directly at the sun and death." Because HIV disease is so linked to death, and because these persons often have many friends who are dying, there is more likelihood of death being faced squarely than there is with other diseases. Once the person begins to talk of death, there is often a feeling of lightness and freedom. A great deal of energy is spent in our culture denying thoughts of death. It is ironic that once death is faced, the person is freer to *live* fully. HIV-infected persons often talk of life having much more meaning after diagnosis than it ever had before. Each moment seems precious, as does each relationship. This is not so true for those dying alone in poverty.

Nevertheless, nurses must be able to accept that these persons will die and must be alert to every hint that they are ready to talk about it. One client told me it made him furious that I had books on death and dying on the same shelf in my office as books on HIV. I asked, "Have you been thinking about dying?" He then spent the rest of the session discussing it.

Support, Caring, and Help of Others

Many people with HIV-related disease become very active in helping others. Part of the reason may be an unconscious "bargain" with God. "If I help others who are less fortunate, I'll be saved." For others it is a form of "do unto others what I would have others do unto me." Still others may feel pressure from peers to get involved. Whatever the reason, those who engage in altruistic behavior benefit in several ways.

First, it normalizes the person's life, providing some schedule and routine. Second, it provides meaning to life. Third, it increases social contacts and creates a social network. While the nurse may help persons get involved in altruistic behaviors, care should be taken not to make people feel guilty if they don't help others.

Rational Suicide

Fearful of a painful death without dignity, HIV-infected persons may want to have a suicide option. For this reason they may keep a lethal dose of pills available. Often, just having this option or having a plan assuages the person's anxiety. The nurse's role when learning of such a plan is a controversial one. Some believe the person has a right to plan "death with dignity." Others believe death should be "in God's hands" only. For these nurses it may be hard to even hear about the HIV-infected person's wish to control death. Some would argue the nurse must listen and try to explore and understand the person's own experience without judgment. Others would argue the nurse must help the person to value and hold on to life.

Chapter 3

Persons in the HIV Spectrum: Late Stage

Dementia

Between 60% and 70% of persons with AIDS eventually suffer some dementia. For many HIV-infected persons who are knowledgeable about the disease, dementia is the consequence they dread most. Some even say they want to commit suicide should it afflict them.

When an HIV-infected person begins to exhibit a dramatic change in behavior a determination must be made whether this unusual behavior results from the HIV acting on brain tissue, the side effects of drugs, or is a result of extreme anxiety. The client I mentioned in Chapter 2 was hospitalized for acute paranoia, then suffered a prolonged, clinical depression. His conditions were not caused by HIV spreading to the brain, and were cleared up with medication and psychotherapy.

Diagnostic Signs

Early signs of central nervous system organicity include the following:

- Confusion
- Forgetfulness
- Difficulty in concentrating
- Slow thinking
- Trouble with balance
- Weakness in the legs
- Behavioral changes
- Apathy
- Withdrawal
- Dysphoric mood

Many of these symptoms, particularly a difficulty in concentrating, apathy, withdrawal, and dysphoric mood, are common reactions to any life-threatening disease, so care is taken to observe for other signs and to conduct further tests.

In the late stages of dementia the following symptoms occur:

- Global cognitive dysfunction (in severe cases)
- Slowed verbal responses or mutism
- Psychomotor retardation
- Wide-eyed stare
- Quiet confusion
- Indifference to illness
- Organic psychosis

- Peripheral neuropathies
- Incontinence
  (Navia, Jordan, & Price, 1986; McArthur, 1987 in Winiarski, 1991)

A battery of neuropsychological tests have been designed to determine whether symptoms result from physical changes or anxiety. Brain scans and examination of spinal fluid are also used to determine whether HIV has invaded the brain and spinal cord. If AIDS-related dementia can be proven to exist, this justifies the AIDS diagnosis, satisfying CDC criteria and making the person eligible for social services and entitlements in many states.

Care

Care of the demented HIV-infected person is not unlike the usual care for persons with dementia or Alzheimer's disease. Because the HIV-infected person with dementia often suffers from early blindness owing to cytomegalovirus (CMV), care takes into account both conditions. Winiarski (1991, pp. 96–97) suggests the following:

1. **Consistency of environment, including how family and friends regard the client, as well as the client's living situation. This is not the time for changes in the patient's "system." If Aunt Rose invites the client for lunch monthly, this should continue. The patient's living quarters should remain stable, with foods kept in their usual positions in cabinets and refrigerator. (A chart of those positions can be posted, if necessary.) If the client keeps an orderly closet and dresser, the order should be maintained.**

2. **Creation and active administration of a "care team," which will help the loved one cope. Team projects may include scheduled visitation, or assignments for regular telephone checks. The primary caregiver could organize friends to call the patient, just to check and to provide reminders (frequency of calls is a judgment of family and the consultant). A fail-safe system should include the possibility of access to the living quarters if the person does not answer an expected phone call.**

3. **Reminder system. Some clinics and doctors write appointments on business cards, but these too often are lost. Clients are encouraged to carry calendars and to note all appointments, or ask physicians' assistants and others to write the appointments into the calendar. Unfortunately appointments are missed because clients fail to consult their calendars. One useful tool is the oversized calendar, posted in the bedroom. The client is urged to transfer appointments from the calendar book to the oversized calendar, and to**

consult it daily or more often. Friends are asked to remind the client whether he consulted the calendar.

4. Adaptation of computer technology and easily available gadgets. More technology is becoming available to remind people of appointments and medications. One useful gadget is the pill box, which can be set to beep at medication time. Other applications clients find helpful are subscriptions to a telephone service that will make reminder calls. Many well-known mail order catalogs advertise goods that, with some creativity, can be used by a neurologically impaired AIDS patient. A recent Hammacher Schlemmer catalog included an alarm clock with a three-inch diameter alarm shut-off button, which can be used by those with motor neuropathies. The catalog has a clock that projects the time in 3-inch high numbers on the ceiling for those with movement or eyesight problems, and a talking pocket watch, made by Seiko, which has a synthesized voice to announce the time. Also, several companies and other groups provide information on disabled persons' use of computers.

5. Reality orientation. Some who have serious dementia may remain socially appropriate but are not oriented to place, time, or circumstance. One hospital patient, awaiting placement in a skilled nursing facility, greeted his visitor by saying he couldn't stay for long, because he had to be at work in 10 minutes. As with the elderly, it is suggested that friends and visitors continue to orient the patient to time, place, and circumstance.

6. A safe environment. This includes monitoring of the person's condition and a willingness to call the physician if any changes occur. This also includes surveying the person's living quarters and removing or locking up any dangerous substances.

7. A realistic outlook at support. Family members and other caregivers must be realistic, both to themselves and to their loved one, regarding what they can provide. Too often, a caregiver will castigate himself for becoming fatigued, irritable, for wanting a respite, for fantasizing escape or even the patient's death. These are natural feelings that accompany caring for a chronically ill and debilitated person. These feelings are exacerbated when a caregiver, for whatever reason, fails to seek respite or otherwise take necessary time off. Caregivers must realistically assess what they can provide, relative to the type of services the person requires. Little is accomplished and all suffer if the impossible is attempted. Consultation with the patient's physician, social worker, or case manager may introduce options, such as long-term care, which may be perceived as abdication, but which in the long run may benefit all.

(From Mark G. Winiarski *Aids-Related Psychotherapy*. Copyright 1991 by Allyn & Bacon. Reprinted by permission.)

DEPENDENCE

As the disease progresses, especially if blindness occurs, HIV-infected persons become more dependent on family, friends, and professional caregivers. The reaction to this dependence varies from person to person. An HIV-infected person's unresolved guilt and self-blame and a caregiver's anger can make a dependent situation much worse. One of my clients became too weak to cook for himself. His wife, who had a great deal of anger toward him, found it hard to help him. She frequently complained he was "milking" the situation for all it was worth. Because he had been dependent and demanding throughout their marriage, it was difficult for her to see his weakness as a result and reality of the illness. Both clients and caregivers may be reluctant to give in to the dependence, for they may see it as just another sign that the illness is progressing. Clients often believe they can prolong their lives by assuming self-care. In some cases such resistance to accepting help can be detrimental. Nurses must find the balance between promoting self-care for as long as it is safe and possible, and helping clients accept assistance when it is finally necessary. The sensitive nurse might say, "I know it's hard for you to accept my help sometimes, but it's O.K."

DISINTEREST

When people reach the final stage of a terminal disease they often begin to withdraw from everyone. They stop calling or writing friends and family and appear to lose interest in the world around them. One client's wife complained, "All he does is sit in that same chair all day. He doesn't even look up when we enter the room."

Dying persons often sleep for long stretches of time. This may be because of the body's need for rest or a result of pain medication, as well as a part of the withdrawal process. One could say that the dying person is withdrawing energy from this world and placing it in the next.

AMBIVALENCE

Experts in death and dying have described the phenomenon of ambivalence in dying patients. Ambivalence stems from the fact that while dying persons know they must give up their loved ones, at the same time they feel abandoned and forsaken by them. This abandonment can be literally true for HIV-infected persons.

Dying persons often feel angry at people who are healthy and have a future. They may try to balance the anger by instead expressing devotion, for example, by clinging to loved ones. A person may be able to die only in the presence of loved ones. In other cases the opposite may occur. There are many accounts of persons dying when others leave the room, after being given "permission" to die. Nurses are sensitive to the ambivalence of the person dying of AIDS. Such a person has so many reasons to be angry. The nurse needs to understand and accept this anger in an empathic way. An appropriate response by the nurse might be, "I know how hard this is for you." The nurse should also remain aware of the patient's need to cling. The nurse's awareness may be expressed as, "I'm here for you. Don't be afraid to ask for anything."

LIFE REVIEW

As HIV-infected persons near death, they often have a tendency to review their lives. These can be relatively short lives, as HIV often infects young people. There are moments that are remembered with pleasure, along with the painful realization that these parts of their lives are over.

At the same time the dying person may also have regrets, such as never having had children or not having the chance to see the children grow up. They may have unfinished business and unresolved relationships.

The nurse can be helpful by listening to the life review and encouraging the expression of any and all feelings. Nurses might also ask if there are friends and relatives still to be called or messages to be sent.

RESOLUTION

As death approaches, the dying person, feeling vulnerable, may finally be able to settle unfinished business and resolve final conflicts. The nurse can help a great deal by allowing the person to accept death. Maggie Callahan and Patricia Kelley, two hospice nurses and authors of *Final Gifts* (1992), refer to this as "preparing to get in line." Dying persons are often visibly relieved when nurses can put the process of dying into words and can help them to talk about accepting death.

NEARING DEATH AWARENESS

Callahan and Kelley (1992) describe four phenomena that occur as the person nears death. These include

1. Preparing for travel or change. Dying people are aware of impending death. They communicate this to loved ones, often using travel metaphors. Examples are asking for a map, asking how the tide is, asking for passports, and so forth. The nurse can be helpful in "translating" this message to loved ones.

2. Being in the presence of someone not alive. The authors give several examples of dying persons seeing and talking with loved ones who have already died. This may be upsetting to family, friends, and caretakers who do not understand, but it is comforting to the dying person. Nurses can be helpful by explaining why the dying person is gesturing, waving, or talking to persons unseen by others in the room. Occasionally others think the dying person is hallucinating or is receiving too much pain medication, or is losing intellectual function. The nurse can help by answering the patient's questions honestly, for example, "Do you know where my mother is?" The nurse replies "Your mother died years ago." When the dying person says "She was just here," rather than argue or humor the person, the nurse replies, "Yes, I understand that you saw her." Often the dying person is visited by someone they do not know has died. In such instances, it is important the dying person be told the truth. The truth can help the person feel comfort at the thought of reunion with the loved one. Lying about the death only leads to discomfort and anxiety.

3. Seeing a place not visible to anyone else. Often the dying person mentions a place no one else can see. It is usually described as lovely, peaceful, and may contain a "light." Often the words "home" or "going home" are mentioned. When this happens the nurse gently asks about that other place or home. "Would you like to tell me about the other place?" "Which home?" "Are you telling us you are ready to leave?" Dying persons are sometimes found on the floor near their beds, perhaps because they have gotten out of bed to follow someone they have seen to the new place.

4. Knowing when death will occur. The dying person often knows when death will occur and communicates this to others. For example, she may say "I won't be here on Sunday." This uncanny awareness, which the authors call "nearing death awareness," is a signal to the nurse and others that loved ones should be called to the bedside for final partings. It is important, therefore, that the nurse hear and understand this message. However, some persons prefer to die alone. They may ask loved ones to go home and rest or go for a walk. They can then die peacefully.

Callahan and Kelley offer a number of practical suggestions for recognizing, understanding, and responding to nearing death awareness.

- Pay attention to *everything* the dying person says. You might want to keep pens and a spiral notebook beside the bed so that anyone can jot down notes about gestures, conversations, or anything out of the ordinary said by the dying person. Talk with one another about these comments and gestures.

- Remember that there may be important messages in *any* communication, however vague or garbled. Not every statement made by a dying person has significance, but heed them all so as not to miss the ones that do.

- Watch for key signs: a glassy-eyed look; the appearance of staring through you; distractedness or secretiveness; seemingly inappropriate smiles or gestures, such as pointing, reaching toward someone or something unseen, or waving when no one is there; efforts to pick at the covers or get out of bed for no apparent reason; agitation or distress at your inability to comprehend something the dying person has tried to say.

- Respond to anything you don't understand with gentle inquiries. "Can you tell me what's happening?" is sometimes a helpful way to initiate this kind of conversation. You might also try saying, "You seem different today. Can you tell me why?"

- Pose questions in open-ended, encouraging terms. For example, if a dying person whose mother is long dead says, "My mother's waiting for me," turn that comment into a question: "Mother's waiting for you?" or "I'm so glad she's close to you. Can you tell me about it?"

- Accept and validate what the dying person tells you. If he says, "I see a beautiful place!" say, "That's wonderful! Can you tell me more about it?" or "I'm so pleased. I can see that it makes you happy," or "I'm so glad you're telling me this. I really want to understand what's happening to you. Can you tell me more?"

- Don't argue or challenge. By saying something like "You couldn't possibly have seen Mother, she's been dead for ten years," you could increase the dying person's frustration and isolation, and run the risk of putting an end to further attempts at communicating.

- Remember that a dying person may employ images from life experiences like work or hobbies. A pilot may talk about getting ready to go for a flight; carry the metaphor forward: "Do you know when it leaves?" or "Is there anyone on the plane you know?" or "Is there anything I can do to help you get ready for takeoff?"

- Be honest about having trouble understanding. One way is to say, "I think you're trying to tell me something important and I'm trying very hard, but I'm just not getting it. I'll keep on trying. Please don't give up on me."

- Don't push. Let the dying control the breadth and depth of the conversation—they may not be able to put their experiences into words; insisting on more talk may frustrate or overwhelm them.
- Avoid instilling a sense of failure in the dying person. If the information is garbled or the delivery impossibly vague, show that you appreciate the effort by saying, "I can see that this is hard for you; I appreciate your trying to share it with me," or "I can see you're getting tired/angry/frustrated. Would it be easier if we talked about this later?" or "Don't worry. We'll keep trying and maybe it will come."
- If you don't know what to say, don't say anything. Sometimes the best response is simply to touch the dying person's hand, or smile and stroke her forehead. Touching gives the very important message "I'm with you." Or you could say, "That's interesting, let me think about it."
- Remember that sometimes the one dying picks an unlikely confidant. Dying people often try to communicate important information to someone who makes them feel safe—who won't get upset or be taken aback by such confidences. If you're an outsider chosen for this role, share the information as gently and completely as possible with the appropriate family members or friends. They may be more familiar with innuendos in a message because they know the person well. (Copyright 1992 by Patricia Kelley and Maggie Callahan. Reprinted by permission of Simon & Schuster, Inc., pp. 213–215)

THE DYING PERSON'S BILL OF RIGHTS

Because death is hard for most of us to face, we may, at times, avoid or even mistreat dying persons. The situation can be even worse for the dying person with HIV because of the stigma and discrimination associated with it. For this reason the "Dying Person's Bill of Rights," which first appeared in *Cancer Care Nursing* (1984), takes on even more meaning for those dying of AIDS. (See Fig. 3-1.)

FIGURE 3-1
THE DYING PERSON'S BILL OF RIGHTS

I have the right to be treated as a living human being until I die.

I have the right to maintain a sense of hopefulness, however changing its focus may be.

I have the right to be cared for by those who can maintain a sense of hopefulness, however changing this might be.

I have the right to express my feelings and emotions about my approaching death in my own way.

I have the right to participate in decisions concerning my care.

I have the right to expect continuing medical and nursing attention even though "cure" goals must be changed to "comfort" goals.

I have the right not to die alone.

I have the right to be free from pain.

I have the right to have my questions answered honestly.

I have the right not to be deceived.

I have the right to have help from and for my family in accepting my death.

I have the right to die in peace and dignity.

I have the right to retain my individuality and not be judged for my decisions, which may be contrary to beliefs of others.

I have the right to discuss and enlarge my religious or spiritual experiences, whatever these may mean to others.

I have the right to expect that the sanctity of the human body will be respected after death.

I have the right to be cared for by caring, sensitive, knowledgeable people who will attempt to understand my needs and will be able to gain some satisfaction in helping me face my death.

Donovan M.I., and Pierce, S.G. *Cancer Care Nursing*. New York: Appleton Century Crofts, 1984.

Group Therapy with HIV-Infected Persons

While many HIV-infected persons enter individual therapy, the majority are treated in groups, usually support groups as opposed to insight-oriented groups. Nurses may act as group leaders. There are a number of reasons why group therapy can be the preferred method of treatment.

First, HIV-infected persons are often abandoned by friends and families. The psychotherapy group often comes to replace the family as a source of support and encouragement.

Second, denial is hard to maintain in an ongoing group of persons who are all infected by HIV. This is one reason why some people resist entering a group.

Third, studies show that people survive trauma and enjoy better physical and mental health if they are able to talk openly about their common concerns. HIV-infected persons who belong to a group have a chance to share their fears and uncertainties, as well as a chance to grow, change, and belong despite daily tribulations and preoccupations. Group members can provide each other with advice and examples of how to live with HIV and maintain control of their lives. Because group psychotherapy reduces stress it may help to slow the progress of AIDS.

In the face of illness and death, there is often a need to search for some existential meaning. As the group progresses, members explore the insults, hurts, insights, and opportunities brought on by AIDS. Group members also have the benefit of belonging to something that will continue to exist after they are gone.

Families are formed in every society for the purpose of passing on traditions, customs, values, and life itself. To the extent that the group comes to represent a family, it can pass on memories of each person after death. "Examples are group jokes inspired by a member, a special kind of altruism extended by another, or an inspirational idea suggested by still another" (Lego, 1993). This legacy may be especially significant for group members who do not have families or who are estranged from their families and for those who are dying alone.

Some HIV-infected persons choose to be in a conventional therapy group, especially if they were in this group prior to infection. Others may opt for conventional individual therapy in addition to group therapy, which may be either insight-oriented or supportive group therapy.

This chapter is adapted from Lego, S. Group therapy with HIV-infected persons and their caregivers. In Kaplan, H.I., Sadock, B.J. (eds.), *Comprehensive group psychotherapy,* 3rd edition. Baltimore: Williams & Wilkens, 1993.

CHARACTERISTICS OF SUPPORT GROUPS

Support groups generally have certain qualities (Rosenberg, 1984) that make them especially conducive to the treatment of HIV-infected persons. These characteristics include homogeneity, a setting for expression or confession, a common language, a horizontal structure, the opportunity for educational and informational exchanges, reality testing, and the development of coping skills.

Homogeneity

Because HIV infection places people in such a unique and at first terrifying situation, it is advantageous to be in a group where others are undergoing the same experience. It is generally considered best to place gays and IV drug users in separate groups, as each homogeneous group has problems and concerns unique to its own population. Groups might also be formed for hemophiliacs, or for HIV-infected women.

Victimization by a System as Opposed to Psychopathology

HIV-infected persons often feel victimized by various systems, including the government, the Federal Drug Administration, the health care system, and the legal system. The group setting provides an opportunity to express anger, share frustrations, and even mobilize action or defense against the victimization.

Public Confession of Qualification for Membership

Many HIV-infected persons have no forum to discuss their health status, their homosexuality or bisexuality, or their drug abuse. While they may feel stigmatized and discriminated against in society, in the group they are neither marginal nor different. They are accepted and belong, not in spite of their status, but rather because of it. The group, then, becomes a secure place to disclose many thoughts, feelings, and actions that have in the past been kept secret.

A Common Language

Groups that are stigmatized often develop a common language. Because of their mutual experiences, they can understand one another in ways that others cannot. This becomes a way of maintaining cohesion and defending themselves against outsiders. In the support group, members can communicate openly and with easy understanding of commonly held problems and struggles.

Horizontal Structure

HIV-infected persons and members of other stigmatized groups are generally not responsive to a "white coat," professionally led group whose leader may be condescending. While no group responds well to this kind of leader, people who feel victimized by society are especially sensitive to authoritarian leadership. Such groups function much better when there is little power-differential between the leader and the members. For example, the leader may be a member of the same population, that is, a gay man or a recovering substance abuser, increasing the chance of understanding the struggles of the group and of developing a common language.

Educational and Informational Exchanges

In support groups of HIV-infected persons, much of the time is spent helping group members learn more about the disease and about staying healthy. Group members can stay well and survive longer if they are well-informed and pro-active in their treatment. Some areas of educational exchange include safer sex practices, the hazards of needle-sharing, wellness practices, and legal issues such as living wills, power of attorney, discrimination, insurance, civil commitment, liability, disability, informed consent, duty to warn or protect, and last wills and testaments.

Reality Testing

One of the advantages of group therapy in any setting is the reality testing it provides. Often group members who are acting out will be pressured by the group to act more rationally. For example, one group member described going to bars and participating in unsafe sex after diagnosis. The group confronted him about the destructiveness of his behavior and helped him express anger; as a result he was able to stop acting out outside the group.

Development of Coping Skills

Support groups help members cope with the problems they share in common as well as those unique to each individual member. For example, a woman was struggling for a way to tell her child that she had AIDS. The group helped her by discussing when the right time might be, who should be present, and what she could say to the child.

GOALS OF GROUP THERAPY

In the course of group therapy, it is hoped that HIV-infected persons will be able to:

1. Accept the illness

2. Express otherwise unacceptable feelings of rage, sadness, jealousy, shame, and guilt

3. Decrease anxiety

4. Regain the ability to manage their lives

5. Reach out to others for practical and emotional support

6. Face the fear of loss and death

7. Increase self-esteem

8. Reduce high-risk behaviors

9. Deal with substance abuse if it is present

10. Find new meaning in life

11. Reconcile with estranged family members

12. Find ways to show concern for significant others who may be overwhelmed by the member's illness

13. Examine the ways they may leave a legacy unique to their own lives (Lego, 1993)

TECHNIQUE

In groups for HIV-infected persons, conventional group therapy technique is modified to meet the unique needs of these members.

Assessment

HIV-infected persons are likely to enter a group after the shock of diagnosis has subsided and they are ready to consider how to best live their lives with HIV. An intake interview is done to explore the person's reasons for entering a group, prior group experiences, acceptance of the diagnosis and initial adjustment, available social supports, current physical capacity, mental status and apparent coping capacity, and anticipated or actual reservations about being in a group with other HIV-infected persons who are ill and may die (Gambe & Getzel, 1989).

Co-leadership

Group co-leadership is recommended as a way to share responsibilities. For example, co-leadership can make it easier for nurses to make follow-up phone calls when members are absent and to visit hospitalized or home-bound members. Co-leadership also provides mutual support and emotional outlets for the group leaders as they identify with the members' tragedy and pain (Gambe & Getzel, 1989; Child & Getzel, 1990).

Group Composition

As with many other groups, a membership of 7 is ideal. The group should not contain more than 10 members, as groups of this size tend to break into subgroups. The group should not have less than 7 members since there may be frequent absences because of illness. If the group is composed of IV drug abusers, the members should also be receiving separate, ongoing individual treatment, if possible (Gambe & Getzel, 1989). It has been recommended that persons with Kaposi's sarcoma (KS) be in their own separate groups, as their prognosis, survival, and complications are much different from those without KS (Spector & Conklin, 1987).

Setting

Sessions should be held in a warm room since HIV-infected persons are often thin and vulnerable to the cold. Smoking is not usually permitted and ventilation should be good so that those recovering from pneumonia have clean air. The setting must allow for access by wheelchairs and intravenous equipment. If sessions are held in a hospital they should be held off the AIDS unit so that patients are not further stigmatized.

Group Process

The first session of a group is the time for the nurses to introduce themselves, describe their professional backgrounds, and tell why they want to work with HIV-infected persons. They mention that they have known many HIV-infected persons, and reassure members that their stories will be understood. In this session it is important to discuss and agree to confidentiality. Members are introduced and tell the group how and when they were diagnosed (Gambe & Getzel, 1989).

Nurses should be supportive, point out underlying themes, and avoid elaborate interpretations. Care is taken to leave control of the group in the hands of the members, as they may feel out of control in other areas of their lives.

As the group progresses, the members focus on coping with the current crises and developing plans for remaining as healthy as possible. As members become comfortable with one another they may begin to discuss their personal lives, looking for common bonds. Often unconscious competition and testing of the nurses occur. Eventually, conflict among the members and transference to the nurses emerge. Group interaction often reveals ambivalence about being cared for and caring for others (Gambe & Getzel, 1989).

One of the curative factors in group psychotherapy is universality (Yalom, 1985). This factor is important in groups of HIV-infected persons because members often feel isolated and alone. In the group they discover that their thoughts, feelings, and actions are similar to those of others. Thoughts or feelings they may have considered unacceptable, such as rivalry for group attention, a greed for life itself, even resentment toward healthy nurses or a secret wish to infect them may be felt to some extent by every group member. Those "bad" or "odd" thoughts come to be seen as a normal part of living with a fatal disease.

Discussions often center on experimental drugs and medical procedures. Subgrouping may divide the group into those who want to return to prediagnosis functioning, and those who view AIDS as an experience from which they will never recover and who are able to talk openly about their own death and the deaths of others (Gambe & Getzel, 1989). The nurses encourage the open expression of feelings, helping to make overt what has been covert (Lego, 1984).

Leadership

Before assuming the leadership of a group of HIV-infected persons, nurses must carefully examine their own personal values and possible bias toward homosexuality or drug use. Also, they must be able to discuss death and dying and be comfortable working with persons whose death may be imminent.

Nurses must be able to avoid dominating the group and let natural leaders emerge as the group moves forward. They must be able to accept and understand highly varied emotions, especially anger and despair, and must be comfortable discussing sex (Spector & Conklin, 1987). They must also be aware of and honest about their own concerns, for example, about being at risk themselves.

Nurses should be highly knowledgeable about AIDS. Knowledge will allow them to clear up any misconceptions the group members may have, to recommend community resources, to monitor the mental states of group members, and to recognize the early signs of central nervous system complications (Spector & Conklin, 1987).

One role of the nurse is to encourage problem solving and self-care so that members can begin to feel they have some control over their lives (Child & Getzel, 1990). In addition, the leader encourages the members to help one another and to reach out to others for help. Unlike some conventional therapy groups in which meetings outside the group are discouraged (Lego, 1984), HIV-infected persons do meet outside the group, since their social isolation is severe (Beckett & Rutan, 1990).

The nurse should report the death of a member to all the other members by telephone as soon as possible. This alleviates members' anxiety about arriving at a session only to learn that a group member died a few days earlier (Beckett & Rutan, 1990). Members are urged to grieve for members who die by talking about them in the group (Tunnell, 1991).

Confidentiality

Confidentiality is of major concern to HIV-infected persons, as the knowledge of the HIV status could lead to the loss of their families, friends, jobs, health insurance, housing, and civil liberties. The nurse is sometimes faced with the "duty to warn" dilemma, such as when HIV-infected persons are having sex with persons who are unaware of their partner's HIV status. Nurses should discuss these confidentiality concerns in the group.

In the case of destructive behavior, an advantage of group therapy is that the members provide not only understanding but peer pressure to encourage the destructive member to act in a responsible way (Posey, 1988). The nurse and the other group members can help members explore their reluctance to inform their partners and others at risk. Alexandra Beckett and Scott Rutan (1990) found that many times the group helped other members exercise self-restraint and altruism.

Other than when a group member's behavior can cause harm to others, confidentiality is carefully guarded by nurses. Group members must also be able to rely on each other to maintain confidentiality. Issues of confidentiality arise when group members accidentally meet in public, when they must leave telephone messages for one another, and when they meet the families and friends of group members (Posey, 1988). The nurse should help group members explore these issues in the context of support and trust.

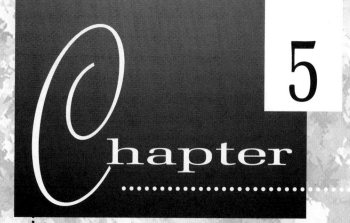

Chapter 5

Families and Friends of Persons in the HIV Spectrum

REACTIONS OF FAMILIES AND FRIENDS

Shock

One of the first reactions of families and friends who learn their loved one is HIV positive is shock. Like the HIV-infected person, loved ones experience bewilderment, and their response is often "Why me?"

Families of gay men or IV drug abusers are doubly shocked if they were unaware of the HIV-infected person's life-style. Parents, for example, may live at a distance, both geographically and emotionally. The shock of this double disclosure may draw them closer, or in some cases increase the chasm.

The nurse involved in professional relationships with families and friends can be helpful by allowing them to express any and all feelings and reactions without passing judgement. A nonjudgmental approach allows "irrational" reactions to come to light. For instance, mothers might say, "How could he be this way? My other children are normal!" or "Am I to blame?"

Guilt about Life-Style

In the case of homosexuality, it is not unusual for family members, especially mothers, to believe they are to blame for their son's homosexuality. The nurse can be helpful by pointing out that blame is not the issue, rather, the primary concern is the HIV-infected person who is in need of support. It is not uncommon for family members to react selfishly at first, focusing on their own hurt or anger. The nurse can gently help them move from this narcissistic position to a more altruistic one.

When the HIV-positive person is an IV drug abuser, family members and friends may feel guilty about enabling the drug use. They may have introduced the person to drugs, given money to buy drugs, or may believe they did not work hard enough to get the person to stop using drugs.

In some cases families and friends have helped keep the life-style of an HIV-positive person a secret. They, too, may feel guilty and responsible for the HIV infection: "If I'd only told my dad, he might have gotten him help! Now it's too late." The nurse can help families and friends by reassuring them they are not responsible for the lives of other adults.

When the HIV-positive person is a teenager or child, parents often experience guilt and remorse. The nurse can help by encouraging open expression, pointing out that parents are not alone, and providing information about support groups.

Fear of Contagion

Sexual partners who learn of their lover's HIV-positive status will fear that they may also be HIV-positive. Testing may follow quickly or, if both partners feel "doomed," may be delayed. The nurse can be helpful by allowing the uninfected partner to sort out feelings and decide what to do, and by presenting the latest information about early treatment.

When families and friends live with an HIV-positive person there may be fear of contagion. The nurse can allay these fears by pointing out that HIV is not transmitted through casual household interactions, but rather through an exchange of body fluids. The nurse can supply literature on avoiding contamination and, equally important, be a supportive listener.

Anger at the HIV-Infected Person

As in all life-threatening diseases, it is very common for loved ones to experience anger at the sick person. There is often a feeling of betrayal, either figuratively, because the sick person is not living up to the irrational contract to live "happily ever after," or literally, in the case of sexual unfaithfulness. Families and friends of HIV-infected persons often believe the persons "brought this on themselves" through the "sin" of homosexuality or drug abuse.

As nurses we can help friends and families understand that behaviors leading to infection can have little to do with will power or right and wrong. When faced with rigid religious or moralistic values, the nurse can avoid arguments and confrontation by saying, "I know you feel hurt and betrayed. That's a natural feeling. It will pass, and eventually you'll be able to help John."

Guilt over the Anger

Because the HIV-infected person may be sick, in pain, and about to die, families and friends may feel guilty about their anger. The nurse can reassure them by explaining that this anger is part of a natural process, and by encouraging them to express and further explore these feelings. Such support and reassurance reduce the chance that the anger and guilt will be expressed toward the HIV-infected person, who is already burdened. In other words, in the context of the nurse-patient relationship, the nurse tries to help people express their individual feelings as well as more common, universal ones.

Survivor Guilt

Survivor guilt is becoming an accepted phenomenon in the gay community. In New York City the Manhattan Center for Living advertised a therapy group for HIV-negative men. The response was so great that *two* groups were formed, and six waiting lists were started. Gay men are confronted with continual loss and grief over the sickness and death of friends. With such a deluge of grief, it is not surprising that those who are spared feel guilty. It is a little like being in a car crash in which all your friends die, and you walk away unscratched. A connected phenomenon is the participation in binges of unsafe sex following the death of a friend. AIDS Project Los Angeles has begun an advertising campaign to combat these lapses into self-destructive behavior. One of their advertisements reads, in part, "When I tested negative, I felt like I had betrayed my friends." Some gay men are reluctant to reveal they are HIV negative and may even lie about it.

How can the nurse help these survivors? As in all cases of anxiety, it is helpful to express any and all feelings. Learning that such guilt is a common phenomenon is also helpful. The nurse can point out that the survivors do not "deserve" to die any more than their friends did. And the nurse should try to help the survivors channel their energy into constructive rather than self-destructive behavior. For example, guilt feelings are sometimes alleviated by helping others or by political action.

Depression

Depression is the most common reaction to loss or anticipated loss. Once the shock, anxiety, and guilt have been weathered, friends and families sink into depression and the beginning of anticipatory grief. If the HIV-infected person is relatively healthy, the depression may be kept in abeyance, but it is never really gone. Friends and families learn to savor happy moments, but the anticipation of sickness and death may linger in the background. The nurse can help by encouraging friends and families to discuss feelings, especially about past losses or anger that may be feeding the depression.

Belief That God Is Punishing Them

It is not uncommon, especially in religious families, for friends and families to believe that HIV is a punishment from God. Plagues have served as a metaphor for God's anger since the beginning of religion.

Such a belief can be especially difficult for nurses to handle. First, because our practice is based on theory and science we may consider the idea of God's revenge to be irrational or ignorant. We must remember that these beliefs are often firmly held and deeply ingrained.

The nurse can help by listening nonjudgmentally. If family and friends sense that the nurse is condescending or hostile, they may turn away and refuse to communicate. When a family member or friend is deeply religious, a chaplain or other spiritual guide can be helpful.

Family and friends may ask nurses about their own religious beliefs and practices. I have found it useful to be honest and open at those times.

Shame

Often, families and friends feel shame about HIV. Susan Sontag, in her monograph *AIDS and Its Metaphors* (1989), talks of her own experience with cancer. She found that fellow patients "evinced disgust at their illness and a kind of shame" (p. 100). Shame in general is differentiated from guilt: guilt is a feeling of remorse over what one has *done;* shame is a feeling of remorse over what one *is.*

Family members of HIV-infected persons sometimes believe that they *are* bad, and that the HIV-infected person is a symbol of this "badness." The nurse can help by pointing out that although we may think that bad things happen to us because we are "bad," there is actually no connection. At the same time we should be careful not to cut off communication with hasty reassurance. It can be very helpful for the person to express any and all thoughts on the subject, no matter how irrational they may sound to us. For example, a patient of mine whose husband is dying recently asked me if she was being punished for a marital infidelity 20 years ago. When I reassured her that there was no connection between these two events she seemed relieved, at least for the moment, and was then able to express her guilt and shame.

Fear of Notoriety

Because of the stigma of HIV, fear of notoriety is not unfounded. Family members, especially parents of HIV-infected children, often are burdened by grief as well as a fear others will learn about the illness. Children may be taunted, teased, and tormented if others learn of their HIV status.

The nurse can help by talking with families and friends about who they wish to tell. The nurse can help them understand that it's okay to keep the HIV status secret to protect them and their loved ones from further distress; it does not mean that this secret is a source of shame.

Social Isolation

When friends and families learn of the HIV status, they may be isolated by their shock. As time passes, there is a desire to move back into social networks. However, a distance now exists between them and others who are not undergoing the same feelings of loss, guilt, shame, and depression.

Stigma also plays a part in the isolation. In her book *AIDS: The Ultimate Challenge*, Kübler-Ross (1987) compares cancer and AIDS. When a friend or family member has cancer, there is overwhelming support. Friends offer comfort, prayers, even food. But when the illness is HIV, there is often only fear or even blame. This places a double burden on family and friends.

The nurse can help alleviate the effects of this isolation, particularly loneliness, by letting stigmatized friends and families know that they are not alone. The nurse can provide an emotional atmosphere of comfort and acceptance. Nurses can also encourage family members and friends to join support groups, where they can talk to others who are undergoing the same painful feelings.

Helplessness

Family and friends often share the same helpless feelings as the HIV-infected person. Those who cope best are those who are able to take a pro-active stance. In *Borrowed Time* (1988), Paul Monette writes about his frantic involvement in learning everything there was to know about AIDS when his lover got sick. He became an expert on the disease, calling friends who were knowledgeable about AIDS, reading, and learning all there was to know. He reduced his anxiety by channeling his energy into productive activity. This, in turn, reduced his feeling of helplessness.

For families and friends, the HIV-positive diagnosis signals a new chapter in their lives. Monette calls this "living on the moon." One of the ways to combat the sense of helplessness during this period is to engage in helping behavior.

The nurse can help by pointing out that there are many things families and friends can do to improve the life of the HIV-infected person. In particular, they should be emotionally as well as literally involved in promoting connectedness with others and wellness behavior. This often requires a great deal of time, energy, and commitment.

Anger at the Health Care Community

From the time the person becomes HIV positive, families and friends become intimately involved with the health care system. This can be very frustrating, especially when there are frequent hospital admissions. Hospitals are often highly bureaucratic, with layers of distressing rules and regulations leading to irritation and anxiety. Staff members are sometimes uninformed, hostile, and insensitive.

The nurse can be helpful by letting families and friends voice their anger. Some of it is justified and some is displaced. With displaced anger, the nurse can help persons identify what they are actually angry about, and reassure them that their anger is a natural part of the process. The nurse might ask, "Of all the things to be angry about, what do you suppose is making you most angry?"

Suicidal Feelings

Upon learning their loved one is HIV positive, families and friends may develop suicidal feelings. In the gay community, people are continually in a state of grief, losing one friend after another. If a man is estranged or distant from his family, has no children, and is losing one friend after another, the knowledge that his lover is HIV positive can be the last straw. Similarly, a woman who has lost a husband or child to AIDS may feel suicidal.

The nurse must be sensitive to the possibility of suicidal thoughts in families and friends. A comment like "I wish God would take me, too. I can't survive without him," or "Without my child there's no reason for me to live," alerts the nurse that the friend or family member may need psychotherapy.

Decline in Sexuality

Friends and spouses often lose interest in sex following diagnosis. The first and obvious reason is the fear of contracting the virus. Decline in libido may also be connected to anxiety, depression, and grief. For the HIV-infected person, sex may be important for life-affirmation or as a means of feeling close to and loved by the partner. If one partner is interested and the other is not, the nurse can be helpful by encouraging the partners to talk openly to one another about their feelings. This may decrease the feelings of rejection and loss each is feeling, and bring the couple emotionally closer.

Conflict

Conflict is a common phenomenon when families or friends are confronting the impending death of a loved one. When the death is HIV-related, the situation becomes even more complex. For example, if the family is distant and the HIV-infected person is gay, conflict may erupt over the person's relationship with his lover. The family may have a difficult time understanding their son or brother's life-style. In the television movie "Andre's Mother," aired on PBS, Sada Thompson plays a mother who arrives in New York to attend her son's memorial service. In a series of flashbacks she reviews her slow, steady recognition over the years that her son is gay and lives with a man. At the memorial service she comes to realize how little she knew of her son, and how much his friends knew and loved him.

Sometimes parents are divided. In the made-for-television movie "An Early Frost," Gena Rowlands and Ben Gazzara play the parents of a gay, HIV-infected young man who comes home to die. At first his father refuses to talk to him, taking a distant, macho stand. But his resolve crumbles as grief overtakes him.

Conflict also occurs between families, friends, and health care providers. Often hospital personnel are not sensitive to visitors. In one instance, a patient was dying, and his lover was stroking and comforting him in his last hours. The nurse became irate and ordered the visitor to leave!

Nurses are often in a position to mediate conflicts. It is important to do so diplomatically and carefully, so neither person feels like the loser. Nurses are most helpful when they remain objective and appreciate the viewpoint of each person involved in the conflict. A nurse who takes sides can make matters worse.

Out-of-Phase Stress

It has often been said that one of the tragedies of HIV is the young age of those who are infected and die. Most often they are young adult men in their twenties and thirties, though the numbers of young women and children are increasing. The emotional pain of the death of one's offspring has been ranked one of the greatest stressors in life. The pain results both from loss of the relationship as well as loss of the legacy parents hoped to leave behind. In addition, parents who are looking forward to retirement or living alone may have their dreams interrupted by the return of a son or daughter or even a grandchild who must be cared for.

One young, female drug abuser was infected by a long-time lover. After his death she moved in with her grandmother. Their life is now chaotic, because the young woman stays out all night, uses drugs, refuses to eat or sleep properly, and even misses her medication, causing her grandmother intense anxiety. Both are in therapy with a nurse who is trying to help each see the other's position.

Despair Because of the Physical and Mental Decline

It is often difficult for friends and families to face the declining health of the loved one. One mother carried around a recent photograph of her son and asked everyone's opinion of how he looked, saying "Doesn't he look healthy?"

If a family member already has an ambivalent relationship with the sick person, the decline can be even harder. One client talked of her brother who was HIV positive and bedridden in her parent's home. Throughout their lives, the relationship between them had been full of conflict. As he became sicker, she said, "He always wants me to touch him! He grabs my hand when I approach the bedside. I never touched him when he was healthy, I certainly don't want to touch him now!" In that session and many more the client explored her anger toward her brother over the years and her guilt about her current feelings. Before he died they became very close.

Often anger or withdrawal are defenses against the despair. The nurse can help by encouraging friends and family members to explore any and all feelings they may have toward the dying person.

Acute Grief and Sometimes Relief at Death

If the dying persons have been sick and in pain for a long time, families and friends may be relieved when they finally die. In this case anticipatory grief has occurred over time, and the families and friends are relatively prepared. Sometimes death comes sooner than expected, catching everyone off guard and precipitating an acute grief reaction.

A study of mothers who cared for their sons until they died revealed an interesting phenomenon: many experienced symptoms of posttraumatic stress disorder in the year following the death (Trice, 1988). This is easily understood, as the mothers had been under unremitting stress for months on end, just like soldiers in battle who experience the same trauma. Susan Sontag (1989) points out that military metaphors are often used in discussions about AIDS, such as "battling the disease." These metaphors are used for visualization, as when the sick person is asked to picture the disease as an enemy to be fought.

The Need for Final Rituals

Funerals and memorial services are important rituals in our society. They provide a last goodbye, an opportunity for openly displayed grief, and a chance for friends and families of the bereaved to show their support and love. This is especially important when stigma is involved. The nurse can help friends and families to plan the service with the HIV-infected person.

The Names Project, also known as the "AIDS Quilt," provides the same function. Loved ones can contribute a panel for the quilt, which travels around the country as a movable monument. The panel is designed to honor the deceased person's life. Friends and families are thereby able to participate in an ongoing public grief ritual and memorial to their loved ones.

SUPPORT GROUPS FOR FAMILIES AND FRIENDS

Support groups help families and friends both during the illness and after the death of loved ones. One of the goals of support groups is to encourage the open expression of feelings. Members may believe they have to be strong in front of the sick person or other family members. The support group may be the only place where people can let down their armor and display feelings they may consider unacceptable, such as anger at the sick person. One wife of an HIV-infected person announced in group, "Bob is up to his usual shit, manipulating everyone to feel sorry for him!"

A second goal of support groups is to support the member's constructive involvement in the care of the sick person. The group helps members find the balance between overdoing care and "infantilizing" the person, and withdrawing because of anger.

Robert Hays (1993), a social psychologist in California, conducted semi-structured interviews of 25 gay men with AIDS, examining their relationships with friends, family members, and caregivers. An analysis of their responses yielded behaviors that are seen as helpful and unhelpful (Fig. 5-1).

FIGURE 5-1
BEHAVIORS OF FRIENDS AND FAMILIES PERCEIVED AS HELPFUL AND UNHELPFUL BY HIV-INFECTED PERSONS

Behaviors perceived as helpful

Providing encouragement and expressing a positive attitude about the PWA's ability to cope with his or her illness or about the possibility of a cure or treatment.

Providing companionship by spending time with the PWA and engaging in social, enjoyable, or relaxing activities.

Expressing love or concern through physical, verbal, and behavioral gestures, and offering to help in any way needed.

Serving as a confidante and listening with empathy and understanding.

Providing information or advice on medical, legal, social, and personal issues.

Acting as a role model with actions and attitudes that inspire and motivate.

Giving the opportunity for reciprocity; letting the PWA feel valuable and needed.

Interacting naturally with the PWA in the same way that one always has.

Providing practical assistance by helping with day-to-day tasks and errands.

Behaviors perceived as unhelpful

Acting patronizing or overprotective and treating the PWA like a child; making decisions for him or her.

Avoiding interaction with the PWA, leaving him or her alone or excluded from social activities.

Avoiding discussion or expression of feelings about AIDS and related emotional issues or acting in an insincere, cheerful manner.

Criticizing the PWA's response to AIDS or giving unsolicited advice on how he or she should act differently.

Acting embarrassed or ashamed and expressing the desire that the PWA hide his or her illness from neighbors, relatives, or others.

Breaking confidentiality—telling others of the PWA's illness without permission.

Making unreasonable demands or being insensitive to the limitations that AIDS places on one's abilities.

Acting in a judgmental manner—making comments that suggest that the PWA is to blame for his or her illness, or using religious and moral references to attempt to change him or her in some way.

FIGURE 5-1 *continued*

Behaviors perceived as helpful	Behaviors perceived as unhelpful
Providing material aid or gifts, which eases the financial strain of AIDS and serves as a gesture of love.	Expressing a pessimistic or hopeless attitude about AIDS or acting gloomy and depressed.
Providing a philosophical perspective and participating with the PWA in exploring spiritual and philosophical meanings of life and illness.	Expressing doubt about the PWA's medical care or questioning the PWA's medical provider's competence or the effectiveness of the medical treatment.
Providing support for other network members, easing the PWA's sense of sadness and/or guilt that his or her illness causes pain or is a burden to his or her loved ones.	Making rude or insensitive comments or actions, such as making fun of symptoms, smoking in his or her presence, or not allowing him or her to be alone.

From *A Message to the HIV Frontline*. #11 Jan./Feb. 1993

The most important goal of support groups is aiding in anticipatory grief. Because all group members are about to lose someone or have lost someone, there is shared support and understanding among members.

The nurse who leads the group should allow the group to set the pace, taking control as needed and helping members to talk about their thoughts, feelings, and actions. Common phenomena should be pointed out to help members feel comfortable with irrational feelings. For example, one member said, "I wish he'd just die and get it over with, so I can move on with my life." Other group members are often sympathetic, confessing that they feel the same way. They may ask the nurse, "Is it normal to think such a thing?" The nurse might reply that this is a common reaction, and ask what other thoughts have occurred along these lines. The atmosphere must allow for total acceptance of any and all thoughts and feelings. If members believe the nurse has a "proper" way to react in mind, spontaneity and honesty will be sacrificed, and members will not benefit from the group or may leave it.

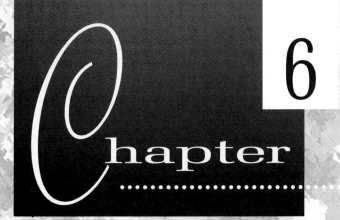

Chapter 6

Professional Caregivers of Persons in the HIV Spectrum

REACTIONS OF PROFESSIONAL CAREGIVERS

The AIDS epidemic has challenged nurses and other health care providers in ways we never could have dreamed. It has forced nurses to look at their own deep-seated feelings about homosexuality, drug abuse, sex, and death. Fears and other reactions to HIV/AIDS are explored in this chapter.

Fear

Although we have a clear picture of how HIV is transmitted, fear often causes nurses to think of HIV as mysterious and "unknown." I have heard nurses say, "They *think* they know how it's spread, but they don't *really* know—maybe it's airborne!" We know that such a reaction, in which scientific knowledge is ignored or downgraded, is the result of a nurse's own fear and denial.

Sophisticated nurses, particularly those who are AIDS experts, understand how HIV is spread and do not fear contagion. While nurses can have a conscious fear of contagion, through needle stick and other concrete, accidental occurrences, they may be masking more subtle, unconscious fears. For example, fear of people with AIDS is often related to the feeling that they are different from "us." If we avoid them, we won't be disturbed by the illicit impulses or "bad things" we think they do, like having pro-miscuous sex or using IV drugs or losing control of their lives. Nurses may avoid HIV-infected persons to avoid or ignore the illicit impulses they represent.

Much has been written about the fear of death. Because many HIV-infected persons are the same age as, or younger than, the nurses caring for them, there is often a "there but for the grace of God go I" reaction. Such fear is especially common when the HIV-infected person shares the nurse's race and gender.

Over-Identification

Occasionally, nurses care for patients with whom they over-identify. Nurses who work on AIDS units in hospitals may see the same person readmitted with each opportunistic infection. The more similarity between the nurse and patient, the greater the tendency to over-identify. One nurse told about a lawyer admitted to her unit: "She was so young and so gifted. The thought of this vital, attractive woman wasting away and dying upset us all." Winiarski, in *AIDS-Related Psychotherapy* (1991), tells of a person he was treating whom he liked very much. When the young man was admitted to the hospital, he did not respond to treatment and quickly declined. Winiarski found himself scanning the chart for something the doctors might have missed and he asked the head nurse to do the same. He suddenly realized he was acting like a worried family member and that he was overly involved in the situation.

Prejudice about Life-Style

A number of studies have shown that many nurses and other health professionals are homophobic. A survey by Douglas, Kalman, and Kalman (1985) of 91 nurses and 37 doctors found that about 10% believed gays who get AIDS are "getting what they deserve" (p. 1,310). About one-third said they felt more negatively about homosexuality since the AIDS epidemic began. Nurses, like the population at large, often have negative opinions about drug abusers and prostitutes.

Increased Anxiety

Many nurses who care for HIV-infected persons report increased anxiety. Nearly all have what Winiarski (1991) calls "The AIDS Dream" (p. 127): a dream that one is suddenly diagnosed as HIV positive or as having AIDS. A variation of this dream is that a loved one is similarly diagnosed.

I first had this dream when I began to lead a support group for AIDS caregivers and heard the heart-breaking stories they told about their patients. While doing research for this book, I often read AIDS-related journals or memoirs in bed before going to sleep. This, too, prompted "the AIDS dream." The dream is a sign that as nurses we are empathetic to the dilemma of our clients. It can be used to examine our feelings about our clients and their experiences.

Increased Negative Ruminations

A study of health care workers who work with HIV-infected persons as well as other patients showed that they ruminated and worried much more when working with the HIV-infected persons (Trieber, F.A., Shaw, D., and Malcolm, R., 1987). These ruminations mostly involved the workers' fear of contracting AIDS or of spreading it to friends and families, and occurred both at work and in nonwork settings.

Negative Perceptions of AIDS Patients

This same study revealed that medical staff had more negative perceptions of AIDS patients than of other patients during routine medical procedures. Nurses have also been found to prefer patients who are not HIV-infected.

Pressure from Friends and Family

Nurses who work with HIV-infected persons may experience not only self-imposed pressure and pressure at work, but also pressure at home. Family members often urge them to move to another field of nursing, worrying that they will contract the virus and pass it on.

One nurse reported that she had a terrible day and had cried at work over a patient. Her mother happened to telephone her when she got home and the nurse told her what a hard day she'd had. Her mother replied, "You have a husband and two beautiful children. Don't you think you should change jobs?"

Despair Caused by a Patient's Decline

The same despair that friends and family members of an HIV-infected person experience is often felt by nurses, especially when they see the same person repeatedly admitted, each time in worse condition. Nurses enter the field to help people get well or stay well. It is painful to watch patients get steadily worse. This is especially true on AIDS units where patients are admitted over and over, each time sicker until they die.

Burnout

Because of continual stress—emotional, work-related, and resulting from family pressures—nurses on inpatient AIDS units often suffer from burnout. I have been told that the average length of stay for a nurse on a well-known AIDS unit in New York City is one year. This probably varies from setting to setting. Similarly, a staff trainer in a home health care agency said nearly all her home health aides quit after the first death.

PSYCHOLOGICAL DEFENSES OF CAREGIVERS

Avoidance

One of the characteristic ways of dealing with anxiety is through avoidance. Many HIV-infected persons have characterized their hospital care by describing nurses who move in and out of the room quickly and efficiently, but who avoid any emotional contact with the person. While they ask questions about the person's IV, catheter, and so forth, they never ask, "How are *you* doing?" One nurse told another, "I get in and out as fast as possible so they can't engage me in conversation."

Denial of Emotional Response

A support group for caregivers was discussing the members' emotional reactions to patients. One remote and distant nurse was asked how he reacts to HIV-infected persons. He answered, "The same as any other patient. I treat all my patients equally." It is likely that the nurse who does not notice any reaction to HIV-infected persons is using denial. Because of all the stresses mentioned previously, it is hard to imagine a caregiver having no reaction. Denial is a way of removing painful, unacceptable feelings from one's conscious awareness.

Sadism

Nurses report that HIV-infected persons are often more angry and demanding than other persons. When this is threatening to nurses they may use their power over these persons in sadistic ways. Kübler-Ross (1987) tells a horrifying story of a prisoner with AIDS who had sores in his mouth. The prison guard, when asked to get him something to eat, brought him taco chips.

Stigmatization

Stigmatization is a way of disassociating oneself from an idea or group that is feared. The stigmatized group is seen as "them" as opposed to "us," creating distance from the feared persons. A nurse who contracted the virus when caring for a patient in the emergency room told of trying to keep her HIV status a secret, though her story was on the wire services and had been broadcast throughout the country. She lived and worked in Iowa. One day a nurse colleague said to her, "Isn't it terrible about that nurse in San Francisco who got AIDS in the emergency room?" She responded, "Why do you say it was in San Francisco?" Her colleague replied, "That's where they have AIDS!" Following this incident the nurse decided to go public about what had happened to her. She decided she could do more good in her campaign to make universal precautions a reality if she helped people see that "them" is "us." AIDS political advocates have praised Arthur Ashe, Magic Johnson, and others who have come forward and "given AIDS a face." The comments of these celebrated figures have helped to reduce the stigma and prejudice associated with the disease.

Over-Intellectualization

Nurses and other health care workers use intellectualization as a frequent defense. It is far easier to talk about the "course of illness," "treatment options," and so forth than to face the feelings of HIV-infected persons, their families, or our own emotional reactions. Nurses sometimes say that to survive they must focus on the illness rather than the person. This attitude is relative; some nurses are far more likely to intellectualize than others.

One nurse spoke of working on a hotline that receives very upsetting calls. For example, a person might call to say he has just learned his lover has AIDS. When this came up in a support group the others asked the nurse how he replied to such a caller. The nurse answered robotically, "To-be-tested-you-may-report-tomorrow-to. . . ." The group accused the nurse of using "canned speeches" to avoid having any emotional involvement with the caller or expressing any feeling. The nurse denied this, saying he was doing his job the way he'd been taught!

Escape into Clinical Details

A defense that is tied to intellectualization is that of escaping into clinical details. I have observed this tendency in support groups as well as conventional psychotherapy groups over the years. Because of this defense, one theory is that leaders of groups of caregivers should not be AIDS experts. When they are, they may have a tendency to slip into the "expert" role, using facts to escape feelings. Of course, another theory is that the leader must be an AIDS expert to effectively help the caregivers.

Self-Righteousness

Another defense against anxiety and anger toward HIV-infected persons is self-righteousness. With this defense, the nurse continually talks about how badly others treat these persons. This "ain't it awful?" diatribe may be seen as a reaction formation: the "others" are acting out in a way this nurse would like to, but does not dare. By repeatedly relating these stories, the nurse attains unconscious satisfaction.

Over-Commitment

A final defense used by caregivers is over-commitment. Examples include working long hours overtime, and feeling guilty when not at work. This might be viewed as yet another variation of reaction formation. Because the nurse is so threatened by HIV-infected persons and the work setting there is a tendency to over-invest. Over-commitment can also be seen as "counter-phobic" behavior. One outcome is that the nurse soon burns out, and leaves the setting without any realization that the defensive behavior was a way to escape the situation. Burnout is seen as a legitimate reason for leaving.

ADDRESSING THE PSYCHOSOCIAL NEEDS OF CAREGIVERS

"Professional caregivers whose work is HIV-related may at times need additional advice, support, or counsel from co-workers or other professionals. Individual counseling or support groups can provide the occasional or continual help that caregivers need."

Individual Counseling

When the nurse becomes anxious to the point of decreased functioning at home or at work, individual counseling may be required. The emphasis is on examining just what in particular is causing the anxiety and what defenses are being used. Counseling can help the nurse to sort out common phenomena from reactions that are idiosyncratic and may relate to other aspects of the nurse's life.

Support Groups

The first goal of support groups for caregivers is catharsis of the feelings of anxiety, anger, guilt, and despair. It is helpful for nurses to learn that these are common phenomena, and do not mean the nurse is "crazy," "mean," or "insensitive." In fact, nurses who recognize these feelings in themselves are more likely to emotionally connect with patients than nurses who are not introspective.

The second goal is to help caregivers notice how they act out these feelings with the HIV-infected person or what defenses they use to protect themselves from these uncomfortable feelings. Again, the knowledge that the feelings are part of common phenomena can help the nurses feel better about themselves.

A third goal is the support and encouragement of one another. In one support group one nurse praised another, telling the group, "She's our clinical specialist. We don't know what we'd do without her!"

And a fourth goal of support groups is the sharing of information about HIV and AIDS. Because our knowledge of the disease is changing so quickly it is helpful to have an informal "clearing house" of information.

In setting up support groups for caregivers, I've found the following practices helpful: First, groups should be held off the unit, even out of the hospital if possible. For example, I found that moving the group from a university setting where we all sat in a classroom on orange plastic chairs to my private psychotherapy office made a big difference. In the comfortable privacy of the office, group members were able to talk more freely than they had in the classroom setting.

Second, groups should be heterogeneous in gender, setting, and discipline. Males may be more able to talk initially, but females may be more comfortable expressing emotion. Each can learn from the other. Differences in setting may make it easier to talk freely and there is less likelihood of complaining about specific people. Heterogeneity in discipline increases the chances of learning.

The first six chapters of this volume have outlined the psychological needs of HIV-infected persons and their caregivers. The next chapter was written by a nurse, Carole Chenitz, who has since died of AIDS. Many of the ideas presented in chapters 1 to 6 are illustrated by her experience both at home and in the hospital.

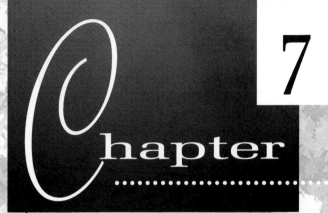

Chapter 7

Living With AIDS

W. Carole Chenitz

In this chapter, I'm going to share my personal experience of living with AIDS. In doing so, I am going to present for the first time to a professional audience my personal life—who I am as a person and as your colleague, and my illness and its impact on me and my family. I will focus on the experience of AIDS for women and look at what nurses have done for me and what they haven't. Finally, I'll take a glimpse into the future, a glimpse that's filled with hope not only for treatment but for change.

Writing this chapter means taking a risk, but I have found that survival with AIDS requires a wellness plan, risk taking, and a willingness and openness to change. I have written a fair amount as a nurse researcher; writing this is different. This is about me, the patient. The patient with a disease that even in 1991 we keep secret. This chapter is not a scholarly work. It is written from the heart to give you a glimpse into the world in which persons with AIDS (PWAs) live.

Even though I am no longer a nurse researcher, old habits die hard. I've therefore included at the end of this chapter a reference list on coping with AIDS and other life-threatening illnesses, as well as a list of books written by PWAs, their family members, and caregivers. (Author's reference list is not included here. For similar information see appendixes and references at the end of this book—S.L.) These lists are meant for nurses and for nurses to give to clients. I find it a great comfort to read others' experiences and I have learned and grown from this reading. Another benefit from reading and hearing about others' experience is that it helps decrease the sense of isolation and increase feelings of empowerment. Self-empowerment is not just a concept or a lofty ideal if one is to live with AIDS; it's got to be a reality. In addition, I've included a resource list of newsletters and sources of information with which nurses and PWAs should be familiar to keep up with the rapid changes in the epidemic. This list is basic to all PWAs.[1]

My family and friends are all I have today. They are what is of value to me now. All the articles and books published, presentations made, studies conducted, classes taught are part of another person in another time. Maybe slowly I'll be able to integrate my professional self with my new self, but that hasn't happened yet. Today I identify myself as a PWA. Making the transition from what *was* in my life to what *is* was difficult. I want to tell you what it's like to make that kind of transition and what it's like to live on the other side of it.

[1]A version of this chapter was presented at the meeting HIV/AIDS: 1990, Hilton Head Island, South Carolina, Nov. 15, 1990. The author thanks Angie Lewis, R.N., M.S., F.A.A.N., for her support and encouragement.

PERSONAL AND PROFESSIONAL BIOGRAPHY

In 1968 I graduated from Kings County Hospital Center School of Nursing in Brooklyn, New York. As a new graduate, I worked in a male trauma unit, the recovery room, and the open heart surgery recovery room. After a year of practice the handwriting was on the wall; if I wanted to make a difference in nursing, I would need a bachelor of science degree. In 1969 I began college, taking a full course load and working full time. In 1970 I married a physician I had met while in nursing school. We moved to South Carolina and then to Boston where we spent several years and had a beautiful baby girl in 1973. The same year I graduated from college. I always worked in nursing, mostly full time.

After moving back to the New York area, my husband and I divorced and I began graduate school. I received a master's degree in psychiatric/mental health nursing from Columbia University in 1976 and a doctorate in education in 1978, also from Columbia. On the doctoral level I focused on research in clinical settings as my functional role. Upon graduation I wanted more training in research methods and was accepted to do a post-doctoral fellowship at the University of California, San Francisco. With my daughter Rebecca, then 5 years old, I moved from the East Coast to the West.

In 1981, upon finishing my fellowship, I began working, first as a nurse researcher/assistant chief of nursing service for psychiatry and then after a year as the associate chief of nursing service for research at the Veterans Administration Medical Center in San Francisco. I stayed at this job until October 1989 when AIDS was diagnosed. I loved my job: my boss was supportive, the nurses were enthusiastic, and I was working in a clinical setting that allowed me to maintain clinical practice and be in touch with patient care.

After my divorce I was involved in a long-term relationship that ended in 1983. After the breakup, I dated a man from May to October 1983. I dated one other fellow before getting remarried in 1987. Life was great. I had a beautiful daughter and was guardian of my precious niece Kim who came to live with us when she was 3 years old.

ON BEING HIV POSITIVE

Two years ago I donated blood during a blood drive. Ninety days later, on a cold, gray, northern California day, I received a certified, registered letter.

It was my day to work the evening shift, as I did every Monday. This enabled me to conduct a seminar for the nurses and to facilitate a multi-family therapy group on the substance abuse inpatient unit. The letter was from the blood bank, informing me that I was HIV positive. My heart stopped as I read the letter. "How can this happen? There must be some mistake. Oh my God, I'm going to die!" I was scared. I felt that I had just walked through a warp in time and space. I was now on the other side of the pale seeing myself and my life as if it belonged to someone else. I felt each breath would be my last. Waves of pain, fear, and sadness washed over me. "What am I going to do? Who can I talk to? What about the children?"

It was time to go to work. I got through the class; I really can't remember any of it except that while I was functioning on one level, I was crying inside. My sorrow was palpable, but I couldn't let it show because I couldn't talk about what was happening to me. I got caught up in the nurses' seminar, and later was able to throw myself into family group and the pain subsided for a brief time.

Within the next 24 hours, I was able to talk to my wonderful husband, two dear friends, and my sister. The support was like a cold glass of spring water on a hot, muggy summer day. It was life giving. They loved me. They were there for me. They didn't feel that I was less of a person, nor were they ashamed of me. Their love, concern, and steady presence enabled me to put one foot in front of the other and take up my path again.

Instead of feeling better, as time passed, irrational fear took hold of me. I was afraid to use the same shower as my husband. I was worried about sharing the soap with him. What about food and kissing? What about when the kids take a sip of the beverage I'm drinking? Now, I was very knowledgeable about AIDS and HIV transmission. I had several dear friends who had AIDS. I never worried about being infected by them, since we did not have intimate contact. Now that I was infected, however, I felt unclean, like a leper, an outcast afraid of infecting someone else. It took several weeks before my rational mind could overcome the irrational fear. As usual, talking about it helped because I was able to share these fears with my husband and friends.

The next week was a blur. I have no idea what happened or what I did. We were scheduled to go on vacation and visit my mother. The kids were really excited, and my husband and I decided that we couldn't cancel but that we weren't ready to talk about it yet. My mother was the last nurse, and she has always been so proud of me. I knew this would cause her incredible pain, and I couldn't hurt her.

I look at pictures from that trip now, and I see this rather typical American-looking family. We're all smiles as befits a family on vacation. That's not how it felt to me. That week was one of the worst in my life. Each step I took, I thought I would walk over the side of the earth. I would look at people and wonder if they knew, if they could tell. I wanted to scream out, "I have the HIV virus!" I wanted to scream, to cry, to hide. Somehow, my husband and I made it through the week. We would whisper about "it" behind our closed bedroom door and then emerge all smiles, ready for the next adventure and fun-filled day.

I decided that I would continue to live life as if nothing had changed. I would not tell people that I was HIV positive until I absolutely had to. Only with a diagnosis of full-blown AIDS would I tell others of my condition. Until then, I wanted to hold onto my life as long as I could. I didn't want my children to be worrying about me when they had their own lives to focus on. I didn't want to cast my AIDS shadow over their lives until it became unavoidable, and until I felt ready in my own heart.

I went into therapy. I cried. I asked, "why me?" I was angry at AIDS, the virus, myself, and my source contact. I was able to get in touch with my sexual partners from the previous decade. They were frightened when they heard why I was calling. Each one except one person called me back. Each said he tested negative for HIV. One person didn't get back to me, and through his family I discovered that his dearest friend had just died of AIDS. Since then we've been in touch, and indeed, he is HIV positive. Even though I was aware of the low rates of transmission from HIV-positive women to their male sexual partners, each phone call terrified me as I worried about whether I infected them or whether they infected me. Was my husband infected too? He tested negative.

Over the next few months my feelings became more stable and I was even able to feel periods of serenity. I constantly had to remind myself that I was okay "today." Sometimes I had to remind myself that I was okay "at this moment." I had to stay focused on the here and now. I've learned that if I get caught up in the past and what I should have done or on the future and what I could do, I start sinking emotionally. In the present moment nothing is ever that bad. So life continued, and I was consciously grateful for every moment.

GETTING A DIAGNOSIS

The American Nurses' Association, Council of Nurse Researchers Conference was in Chicago in September 1989. At the meeting I had a poster presentation. It was, as usual, an exciting, packed meeting with lots of good sessions to attend, old friends to see, new people to meet. During the meeting I was very tired. I had three cups of coffee during the poster session, which was unusual since one cup a day was my limit. Even with the coffee I was tired. I napped frequently, but other than fatigue I felt fine. I went to the Art Institute of Chicago, one of my very favorite museums. We went to a show. All in all, a productive and enjoyable meeting.

Upon returning home I found the usual pile of mail, phone messages, and things to do that had accumulated while I was gone. The week went by quickly. On Friday, after work, Kim had an appointment with her pediatrician for a routine physical. I took her there, and when we came home I was beat. My family rallied and got dinner. The next morning I couldn't get out of bed to take Kim to her swimming lesson. I felt like I had the flu and spent the weekend in bed. On Monday I was still weak but feeling much better. I stayed home from work and at my husband's insistence went in to see my physician.

The physical was fine, my lungs sounded clear, and I was ready to leave. My doctor stopped me. "Carole, as long as you're here, let's get a chest x-ray." I agreed with that, why not? The x-ray was ready within minutes, and we both looked at it. My physician, a young, bright, funny guy, turned to me with grim eyes. There was no laughter in his voice. "Carole, this is scary. Do you see what I see?" I did. Both lungs and both upper lobes were affected. Tuberculosis (TB) or Pneumocystis pneumonia? "You're going into the hospital right now. We need to get a sputum and if we can't get that we need a bronchoscopy."

Bronchoscopy produced a diagnosis, but I could not bounce back from the sedation. I started on intravenous (IV) Septra, but I continued to get worse. The most difficult thing to deal with was being unable to breathe. Even with oxygen it was difficult to get enough air. I was sleepy and had chills and fever. I was acutely ill, scared, trying to hold a front for my children, and feeling a deep sense of despair.

No one is ever prepared for an AIDS diagnosis. There is no way to describe the feelings I had when my doctor said with tears in his eyes, "The bronchoscopy report confirms Pneumocystis. Carole, you now have AIDS." Again, I started operating on two levels. I was chatting with my doctor about treatment while inside I was screaming, "No, no, not me. This is a big mistake. This can't be happening to me. God, help me." Fear, sorrow, and anger swept through me. I just wanted to pull the covers up over my head and pretend it wasn't happening. I felt dirty, damaged, *devalued, a diminished person.* I hated the body that was betraying me. I hated myself. I didn't want to die, but I didn't see how I could live.

MY NURSING CARE

Upon entering the hospital I was placed on TB precautions, and that unfortunately really alienated me from the nursing staff. The nurses would scold my children into wearing masks, keeping off the bed, and the like. It seemed to me that for these nurses the form was critically important. That is, they cared more about whether all of the rules were complied with, whether I had the blanket I needed when I rang the call bell, whether my bed was neat and clean, whether I had the oxygen at the proper setting, and not at all about how I was. I was a case, not a person. Shocked and emotionally distraught about my AIDS diagnosis, this dispassionate care fed my sense of unreality. I was in a living nightmare.

I don't know if the nurses felt intimidated by me. I remember one very young nurse was in the room and my doctor came in with, "Good afternoon, Dr. Chenitz." I responded by using his "doctor" title and we joked and laughed for a few minutes. I glanced at the nurse and smiled. She looked frightened and uncomfortable and left the room immediately. Up until that point I had no idea that I might have a chilling effect on the nurses who cared for me. Since I have always identified as a nurse, I feel at home wherever there are other nurses. We share more than a profession; we share a value system and a way of seeing the world. So, I had never thought that my AIDS diagnosis and who I was (a successful nurse) could frighten other nurses. Whatever the reason, when I needed these nurses, they simply weren't there, but my nursing admission interview was done and I'd wager that my nursing care plan was up to date.

Certainly the nurses were polite, respectful, and nice. But no one ever asked me how I felt. The lonely evenings after my family and friends left were very hard for me. The bed was uncomfortable (with that hard plastic ticking that protects hospital mattresses). My fevers would spike and the night would just seem to come down on me. What was to become of my life? What was to become of my children? What was left? How many more hospitalizations would there be? Would I lose my dignity, self-control, eyesight, ability to think? Would my children be forced to see their mother like that? Should I commit suicide?

Every evening I was tormented, and the nights in hospital became what St. John of the Cross called "dark nights of the soul."

I really couldn't talk to my family and friends about this, since they had enough to deal with. I just couldn't burden them with any more. Sadly, through all this, no one in the hospital stopped to ask me how I felt, how I was. They did their job efficiently and moved on.

Not only did the emotional needs I had go unrecognized, but no one touched me. No one in the hospital staff took my hand, rubbed my back, gave me support, or did any of the comfort and care measures that we nurses pride ourselves on. I will never forget how I felt.

Moreover, the effect this had on me was to be overwhelmed with my body. I was unclean, untouchable, undesirable, a patient with a disgusting disease. If you get too close, you may get it, too. Obviously if I were in good health, in my usual role, and felt like me, this uncaring care would have affected me, but I was now a person with AIDS. I had crossed from caregiver to care recipient. My choice was to accept this role and go on or to sink into the morass that I felt all around me. Oh, how much easier it would have been if one of these nurses had reached out with a warm hand.

Two things happened for me about this time. The first was an answer to my struggle with the question, "Why me?" One night the answer became crystal clear: "Why *not* me?" Illness, tragedy, and misfortune can happen to anyone. I was not immune. I had a good life, and I could still have a good life. So, why not me?

A little miracle also occurred about this time, several days into my hospital stay. A nurse came into my room with flowers. She was the discharge planner and had seen my name on the hospital list with the diagnosis. She had heard me speak at a conference and came to tell me how sorry she was about my illness. She told me I had given a great talk when she heard me she was very impressed. She gave me the flowers and left. I never saw her again. I don't know what you would call her, but I called her an angel. All of a sudden, I was a person again, I had a history. I was someone. It felt so good to be recognized as the old me again.

The emotional impact of an AIDS diagnosis is compounded by the acute physical illness of the person receiving it. For me, it was the sickest I had ever been in my adult life. My defenses were down, and I was concentrating on maintaining bodily functions. I wasn't improving with Septra. I was vomiting, my liver enzymes were markedly elevated, and I was becoming increasingly lethargic. My shortness of breath was becoming worse, and I was now so weak, I couldn't make it to the bathroom. I was allergic to Septra, and started on IV pentamidine. I improved almost immediately. After 5 days, which seemed like eternity, I went home.

Home. What a lovely word. I sat on my couch, looking out the picture window at the grove of redwoods in our yard. The sky was that brilliant robin's-egg blue; white clouds were racing by, chased by the wind. I sat there overwhelmed with gratitude at the beauty around me and that I was here to see it. I gave a silent prayer of thanks for this day, for this image, and for my life. Tears came to my eyes at how beautiful everything is, how beautiful life is.

However, things got bad again and very quickly. I couldn't stop vomiting, and nothing touched the diarrhea. I was getting dehydrated. I couldn't keep an IV in, and it was getting increasingly difficult to find a vein. I have very small, frail veins, and only one on one arm is really usable. The others are too small and collapse easily. Another hospitalization was arranged, this time for a venous access device.

It had now been $1\frac{1}{2}$ weeks since my AIDS diagnosis. I was very sick again and back in the hospital. I was still struggling with what it meant to be a person with AIDS. I still felt unclean and untouchable. I was discouraged, and my lack of control over my bowels was a source of deep humiliation. I was readmitted to the same hospital but to a different unit. This unit was a "healing place" created by the nurses who worked there.

I believe now that these nurses saved my life. I was in bed shortly after admission. It was early evening. I was getting an infusion of blood and waiting for an operating room to open up. I couldn't make it to the bathroom. I just couldn't negotiate the IV pole and my body. I was so weak that any movement was a supreme effort. The bathroom was in Europe and I didn't have a plane. Diarrhea was everywhere. I wanted to die. I loathed myself. Further, my bodily fluids were dangerous to others. How could I put others at risk? I put on the call bell, fighting back the tears.

In came Inge, middle-aged, blond, composed, with a warm smile. "What's the matter?" she asked kindly. I could feel the compassion in her voice. It made me want to cry, but that would be too much for me. "I'm sorry but I couldn't make it to the bathroom. My bed is a mess. I am so sorry."

"What's there to be sorry about? I'll have it cleaned up in a few minutes. You should have a bedpan or a commode near you. Do you think you could make it to a commode by the bed?" I wasn't sure, so we decided I would get a bedside commode and a bedpan in my bed to hold on to for security. Then we both laughed. She turned to leave the room. Suddenly she turned around and looked into my eyes. She said gently, "All your life you have cared for people, now let us take care of you. It's your turn. It's okay, that's what we do. Let us take care of you for a while."

Simple words from an ordinary woman, but they were magic. All the nurses on this unit were like that. They loved being nurses, and they defined nursing as caring, compassionate, loving, nonjudgmental care. They cleaned, bathed, touched, started IVs, helped me to the commode, and gave me medicine with great efficiency, but what really mattered is that they did it with compassion. I felt my sense of dignity return, the dignity I felt in their care. The unit was a healing place where I knew I would live and be okay. I got a glimmer that there is life after AIDS.

The trip to the operating room was uneventful. I returned to my room receiving fluid infusions through my new Groshong catheter. After a tearful good-bye to my nurses, I went home to put the pieces of my life together, which I was ready to do after my time in the "healing place." My healing had begun.

PEER SUPPORT

I needed other people with AIDS. I needed to identify with others and find role models and mentors in my new life. I called around and joined a support group at the Center for Attitudinal Healing in Tiburon, California, which fortunately was close to my home. It was a group for women with HIV and AIDS. I made an appointment with the local AIDS agency, Marin AIDS Support Network (MASN), and started ordering newsletters such as the one from Project Inform, the PWA Coalition Newsletter, and AIDS Treatment News. I had to surround myself with and become friends with people who have AIDS. I wanted to be around people who understood what was happening to me.

The support group has about 30 women enrolled, and six to seven come on an average week. Interestingly, we are all upper-middle-class and middle-class white women. The group members represent the various professions and a range of occupations. These women are essential to my well-being, and today I count some of my dearest friends among the members of the group. If something happens to one of us, we all know and we are all affected. When I am discouraged, angry, or scared, the women in my group are there either on the phone or in person. We fill each other in on the treatment of the month; we share treatment recipes the way other women share food recipes. We meet weekly, and I try never to miss it. I speak to several group members during the week. I feel so blessed to have this wonderful group of women through whom I was able to let go of my professional identity and assume my identity as a woman living with AIDS.

I am connected with the Marin AIDS Support Network, our local AIDS agency. I had never been a client in a social service agency. I was always on the provider side. Now, I was the client. I went for my intake interview. It was very difficult for me to reach out and ask for help. When I did, wonderful people were there to help me across the chasm from what was to what is.

Michael, my counselor at MASN, is one of them. Michael is tall, blond, handsome, and full of information about services and things I need to consider. As my intake interview was ending, I was getting ready to leave when Michael quietly asked, "Carole, how are you dealing with your disability?"

I whirled around. "My what?" I felt angry. I didn't look like I had AIDS. No one could see my Groshong catheter. "What disability?" I responded coldly.

He looked at me steadily. "The fact that you can no longer do the things you once could. It is one of the biggest problems that people I see with AIDS have."

I felt my breath leave me. I had not articulated this, but it was an issue I was grappling with. That was it: I couldn't do the things I once could. I was too fatigued. I had no stamina. I became upset and unnerved quickly. Was this disability? I was so relieved that my struggle had a name. I had been striving to return to the way things were. I had wanted my old life back, although I knew things would never be the same. I had wanted to be the person I once was and to do the things that person could do. That was impossible now, and I had to discover what I could do. This was a whole new ball game, and I couldn't play by the old rules.

The support group members and Michael's insightful and sensitive words provided the context for change and a new life. My family and friends provided the opportunity to change with their loving support and acceptance. I began to see myself as a person with AIDS. I began to accept who I was. I started to enjoy my new life, which centers around my wellness program (Table 7-1), my family, my friends, and my community. Love is the basic operating principle in my life. Those who can't give it or who are living in fear have no place in my life today.

I developed a protective denial. That is, when I am feeling good, I live as fully as I can. I do everything my energy will allow. I don't ignore AIDS, but I don't dwell on it either. I focus on the wellness and what I can do,

TABLE 7-1
PERSONAL WELLNESS PROGRAM

1. Have contact with at least one person with HIV or AIDS each day.
2. Read articles, newsletters, books, and pamphlets to keep informed about AIDS information and treatment.
3. Start each day with prayer and pray several times a day.
4. Have quiet time each day just to sit and be still.
5. Remember my priorities. Don't let the little things bother me.
6. Avoid people who are not loving and supportive. Cut them off and out of my life.
7. Have family time each day.
8. Take time for periods of introspection, such as retreats for persons with AIDS (PWAs).
9. Talk about AIDS to schoolchildren, high school students, and community groups both for disease prevention and to give a face to the epidemic.
10. Volunteer in the community. Help others whenever I can.
11. See friends. "Do lunch" at least once a week with a friend.
12. Try creative projects.
13. Exercise when possible.
14. Go to a physician at any sign or symptom of illness.
15. Follow information on clinical trials.
16. Participate in clinical trials whenever possible.
17. Go to a chiropractor for adjustment at least twice a month.
18. Attend support groups for PWAs.

rather than my illness and what I can't do. On bad days I become more identified with my body. I focus on just getting through the day. I allow myself to watch television (I didn't have a television in my house for 10 years), stay in bed, read, or just sleep. This was unthinkable to me a year ago. During the bad times I consciously work at remembering that nothing lasts forever. All pain stops. All things pass, the bad times as well as the good times.

DISCLOSURE

While I was putting my internal life together, other things had to be dealt with. One of the first questions that a person with AIDS has to answer is whom to tell, when to tell, and how to tell. People were naturally concerned about what I had. Friends and colleagues were calling, sending cards and flowers, and bringing food to the house. Neighbors and parents of the children's friends wanted to know what I had and when I would be able to work again.

The central question was, "Do I tell them I have AIDS?" Or do I simply say, "I had pneumonia" and leave it at that? If I tell my friends and colleagues, could one of them inadvertently slip and tell my children? I could just hear the conversation, "Hello, Becky, this is Marie. I just heard the news about your Mom and I'm really sorry that she has AIDS. . . ."

I knew I had to tell my children. Should I just tell Becky, who was now 16, or should I also tell Kim, now 10? Was Kim too young to know?

What would it do to her emotionally? In any event the hospital did not seem the best place to tell them and I wasn't in any shape to help them through their process. I decided I needed a professional's help with the decisions of if, when, and how I should tell my children. In the San Francisco Bay area, resources are available to deal with all aspects of AIDS. I found an agency that specialized in family issues and AIDS.

As a result of consultation with staff in this agency and my therapist, my husband and I made a plan to tell the children. We would take them away for a weekend; we would not tell them at home where they could be distracted. We would answer each and every question, including how I was infected, as honestly and as completely as possible. The weekend was heartbreaking but drew us all closer together. Both of my children have continued to grow and blossom, even with the knowledge of my AIDS. They have made a conscious decision to live one day at a time.

Becky was writing her college applications, and she was able to answer the question, "Describe a significant event in your life and how it has affected you" by describing finding out that her mother had AIDS and what that meant to her. It was a moving, honest essay. She was also able to tell her favorite teacher, her drama teacher. This woman was magnificent and made it safe for Becky to be open with her classmates. Becky found her friends and classmates supportive and loving.

We were very worried about Kimberly and didn't want her to share my diagnosis with her friends. She wasn't ready to, either. Children in the fourth grade can be mean. We were afraid that if people found out that I had AIDS, Kimberly would be ostracized by her classmates. So we decided to wait. Kim felt comfortable with this, since many of her classmates had made negative comments about gays and people with AIDS. While we were sure that the overwhelming majority of people in our community would respond with concern and compassion, we were afraid about the one or two who would react from unbridled fear.

Once the children knew my diagnosis, I was much more comfortable. The pressure to keep the secret from them was gone. We were able once again to talk openly, which had always been a family value. The evening dinner is a time for getting together and sharing both major and minor events of the day. We could now talk about experimental treatments for AIDS, my latest blood report, political issues surrounding AIDS, and anything else related to my illness. We were a family again.

After this hurdle was cleared, I was free to tell others. I knew I didn't want to return to work. I did not feel physically and emotionally able to handle it. So, I had to tell my boss, another heartbreakingly difficult task. She had hired me 8 years before to create a research environment within nursing service. More than that, we had agreed that the research program had to exist within an academic context. Therefore academic values needed to be part of nursing service values. We wanted nurses to feel the satisfaction of publishing their ideas, conducting clinical studies, utilizing research, reading journals, participating as presenters at conferences and workshops, and so forth. For 8 years my boss supported me in this effort. Without her there could be no research or an environment for research in our setting. Further, I cared deeply about her as a person. Telling her would be like telling a family member.

After I was home for several weeks, we arranged a time to meet. It was difficult to tell her because I knew it would hurt her. I received her love, and like the administrator she is, she told me not to worry about ongoing activities. We discussed these, and she took care of them as efficiently as she ran her service. What a gift to me! What a relief! I could go back and clean out my office, but I didn't have to see a lot of people and talk about what was happening.

It was still a shock to me that my life was evolving this way. Initially I was too sick to think about my life and my goals. Later, when my energy was so low, loss of work wasn't difficult to bear, since I couldn't do it anyway. However, the loss of who I was and what I had done my entire adult life, hit after several months: I wasn't a nurse anymore. I still had a license, but I would never practice nursing again. All of the articles published, papers presented, book chapters written, grants developed, and classes taught didn't matter now. It was gone. If I were to survive, I would need to develop new skills. I would have to learn to accept my new life. I needed to learn to relax. Maybe I could salvage something from my old life, but I wasn't sure what.

WOMEN WITH AIDS

All people with AIDS experience, to a greater or lesser degree, physical, social, emotional, and economic changes as a result of the disease. This common shared experience creates a bond between us and is felt in support groups, meetings, parties, or wherever two or more people with AIDS meet. The major group affected by AIDS has been men, particularly gay men. Women, while not newcomers in the epidemic, are sadly taking our place among the groups hard hit by this disease. In my experience and those of the women I know, several issues make this experience different for women than it is for men.

The first and perhaps most difficult issue for women is related to our children and childbearing. Almost every woman I know, if she has children, asks, "What's going to happen to my children?" Fear for our children and the stigma they may have to bear keeps us silent and invisible. The desire to maintain a normal family life, however that is defined, makes us hesitate to tell them. In addition, the long protracted illness affects them deeply, and we know it but are powerless. The sense of frustration at our inability to fulfill the maternal role can lead to despair.

For many women who have not yet had children, the mourning is for the loss of this dream. The biological clock has wound down, yet they are only 24 or 29 or 33 years old. They will never experience the joys of pregnancy, childbearing, and motherhood. Other women decide to have a baby in spite of their HIV-positive status. These women may be judged harshly by others and treated with disdain and scorn by health care providers. "How dare she have a baby when she's HIV positive? Doesn't she know what she's doing? She could infect her own baby." Even other PWAs criticize the decision to have a baby under these conditions. For some women, however, having a child is the fulfillment not only of a life's goal but also of their identity. Who are we to judge?

Another issue that faces women is the curiosity factor. When people find out I have AIDS, the first thing they ask is, "How did you get it?" People presume that they know how a man was infected. However, with women, especially white middle-class women who don't fit some stereotype of PWAs, there's a tremendous sense of curiosity.

I expect curiosity from the community but not from health care providers. I have gotten to the point that I ask for the clinical relevance of this question. "Is my source of infection going to affect my care? If not, then you have no need to know." While this might seem rude, I think satisfying one's curiosity is rude. I am a very personal and private person. I have always been reticent about discussing my sexual life with anyone other than very dear friends. Since I have AIDS, there is an assumption that I am willing to discuss my past and present sexual activities with all comers. I find this assumption offensive. I know many PWAs who don't feel this way, who feel quite comfortable discussing their personal sexual lives, but I'm not like them. Each PWA is a unique person with his or her own world view and reaction to the disease.

Access to information in the AIDS epidemic is lifesaving. Information about treatments and experimental drugs or clinical trials to prevent opportunistic infections, such as clofazimine to prevent *Mycobacterium avium-intracellulare* infection, is critical. Information gives us the essential facts upon which to make decisions and to act. Without information the individual has very few options for treatment.

The gay community has been very effective at mobilizing in the epidemic. Information about treatments and experimental drugs and clinical trials can be found within this community. Women, however, have two handicaps: we are not part of the community, and many of us do not have the educational background to understand what we need to know or how to access this critical information. The gay community was open, sharing, caring, and positive when I initially made my contacts as a PWA. A woman must be proactive, however. If you are not part of the community in which this information is commonplace, you must seek it out. I spend hours every week on AIDS health care news. I wonder with great concern how women without my resources and knowledge manage to get and assimilate this information.

The final issue that women confront is the lack of knowledge about the effects of the virus or the treatments on women. While all PWAs face the overall lack of knowledge and lack of treatments, for women the situation is even more abysmal. There is a recent movement to have the Centers for Disease Control's definition of AIDS changed to include the vaginal and uterine infections that women manifest. This is only one of the issues.

Clearly, discrimination against women exists in the enrollment in research projects and clinical trials. The excuse is that participation in research is too risky because women bear children. A woman's word that she is not going to have a child is not enough. If a woman is enrolled and her reaction is different from the others', there is no way to know if the reason is the treatment under study or the virus. Even basic natural history data on women is lacking. The much talked about findings that women with AIDS die sooner may or may not be true in all populations of women, but this remains to be seen. We have so many questions and so few answers.

THE FUTURE

As I look toward the future, I have no doubt that AIDS has changed and will continue to change health care. In the future I believe several things will happen in relation to AIDS and health care.

First, there will be an end to what I call therapeutic nihilism. This attitude of health care professionals is characterized by a lack of assertive or aggressive treatment for PWAs. For some providers it's a form of burnout. They have had so many people die, they no longer have the drive to seek out experimental treatments or to be creative about treatments. For others, it's a way to withdraw and not deal with AIDS. Therapeutic nihilism toward persons with AIDS is demonstrated by providers who ignore minor symptoms: "Don't worry about hair loss (or fungal infections on the feet or face rash or missed menses). At least you're alive and this won't kill you." Another form is, "So what are you worrying about, you're going to die anyway." A more subtle form is not to find out about new treatments. If the treatment doesn't work, that's it.

I believe therapeutic nihilism also manifests itself in the standard treatment of persons who are HIV infected but without symptoms. The standard is to wait until the numbers of T4-helper cells drop to a certain point and then to initiate treatment. This attitude allows people to be at high risk before treatment is initiated. Once the T4-helper cell numbers start dropping, I haven't heard of anyone who has been able to restore them to a normal or near normal level for any significant period of time. Why are we waiting for treatment? Immune enhancers should be started immediately. Low-dose antivirals for HIV-infected people with high T4-helper cell counts are being investigated, and should be. New methods to prevent Pneumocystis pneumonia and other opportunistic infections need to be tested and used. It is simply not enough to tell people to wait until they are at risk before treatment is begun. That's not treatment, that's a death sentence.

Second, our attitude toward death and dying will change. Like many people with AIDS, I am not afraid of death, I am afraid of dying. The dying process and how that will be handled is of great concern to me. Everyone is going to die. Death is a part of life. However, AIDS brings with it a terribly painful, often humiliating dying process and that terrifies me. Compassion, assurance, and competence are what I need from health care providers. You have not failed me if I die. You have failed me if I die alone, frightened, in pain or distress. It is enlightened help with the dying that I need. I want to help maintain my dignity, keep pain free, and allow my family and friends to be there. Too often today this type of treatment is not available. Why not? This is nursing care, and for this we are responsible.

Third, the future in health care is a shared partnership in care. Nurses have talked about a partnership with patients for years, but now PWAs and people with other life-threatening illnesses are demanding partnerships. PWAs have organized into highly effective, vocal political lobbies. The generation most affected by AIDS is the baby-boomers and those who came after. These are not passive recipients of care. They are demanding partnerships at all levels of the health care delivery system: individual providers, the experts at local, state, and national levels, drug companies, the Food and Drug Administration, and the National Institutes of Health. The long time lag from laboratory testing of new therapeutic agents through the several phases of human testing through data analysis and review to final approval is not acceptable to people whose lives may be extended by these agents. PWAs are demanding representation at all levels of decision making about new treatments and the process for approval of treatments.

It has become clear that the system is not trustworthy. For example, in May 1990 a panel of 16 experts was convened by the National Institute of Allergy and Infectious Diseases to determine whether steroids should be used in the treatment of Pneumocystis pneumonia, a major killer of PWAs. They reviewed five unpublished papers whose authors were panel members and reached a conclusion. They then delayed announcing their conclusion until some of the papers had been accepted for publication 5 months later (*San Francisco Chronicle*, 1990). How many people died as the result of this delay? Our lives for their publications. There is something wrong with this system. This type of delay cannot be tolerated when you are dealing with my life and that of others.

In spite of efforts to refute these charges, the foot dragging of federal agencies in approving drugs for use in AIDS care has eroded confidence in the system. To date, 11 years into the epidemic, there is one approved drug to treat AIDS, that is, zidovudine (AZT). Two other promising drugs, didanosine (DDI) and dideoxycitidine (DDC), await review for approval. Six months ago it was evident that I had to discontinue AZT. I was lucky to begin a clinical trial with DDC. How many others are not so lucky? I know many people who can no longer tolerate AZT and have developed neuropathy on DDI or DDC. What antivirals are left to them? Today, there is nothing else in mainstream medicine.

Fourth, AIDS will become a truly chronic disease. AIDS will be the cancer of the next decade. In recent times there has been a great deal of excitement about the prolongation of life in PWAs. Unfortunately, the average life expectancy for PWAs has increased by only 6 months for men. No one is sure about women, since we are so rarely studied.

There is also a danger that we as a society will trivialize the disease. While on one hand we need to eliminate the irrational fear that surrounds AIDS, we need to replace this fear with personal caution and concerned, attentive care. If the disease is trivialized, PWAs will be ignored as they once were by all levels of government and the public, and the virus will spread.

As AIDS becomes more chronic, fear about the virus, the illness, and PWAs will decrease. PWAs will be treated with compassion and concern by all people. The horrible stories of job loss, rejection by family and friends, house burning, and so forth will be a thing of the past.

CONCLUSION

At this writing I have lived with AIDS for 16 months. I have been very fortunate and had not needed to be re-hospitalized, nor have I had another opportunistic infection. I have made the transition from my old life as a nurse researcher to my new life as a person with AIDS. Rebecca is now a freshman in college, and our phone bills are enormous as we call each other. I am a volunteer in Kim's school at the lunch bar and a co-leader for her Girl Scout troop.

On December 1, 1990, I appeared with the mayor of San Francisco at a press conference to commemorate World AIDS Day. I used my name and appeared on local TV and radio news. The word was out in our community, and so far, aside from a few ripples of fear-based concern, the response has been wonderful. The most common thing I hear is, "If there is anything I can do, let me know." This just warms my heart. Kim has had no problems at school; and both the principal and her teacher are watching out for her, but I think our fears were needless.

Periodically, when I least expect it, I feel the pangs of loss and grief: loss of my old life, my goals, my health, even my body, and grief over the loss I continue to experience. My energy never returned to my pre-illness level, and I have to be cautious about my schedule. I do a fair amount of public speaking at schools and community groups, and I find it exhilarating, scary, and exhausting. I do it because it's my way to contribute to the community. I believe that no one should be infected with this virus in 1991. That means we must reach the groups that are getting infected: women and IV drug users. In addition, there is still the need to give the epidemic a face and to inform people that we are human, too, that we are part of the community.

I follow treatment news and experimental drug news closely. After 10 months, AZT was no longer effective and my T4-helper cells continue to decline. I have been on an experimental antiviral for 4 months now and it doesn't seem to be working. This week, I had four T4 cells per cubic millimeter. We are going to have to make some decisions about treatment again. Each time there's a treatment decision to make I am afraid, but the fear passes. My physician is my partner, and we will negotiate another mutually agreeable plan, in spite of the lack of options. I am truly taking each day one day at a time.

PWAs, individually and collectively, are symbolic representations of society's guilt about sex and moral outrage at certain behaviors (Levine & Ram Dass, 1986). We are modern-day lepers, the outcasts, the outsiders. When you care for one PWA, you are symbolically caring for all of us. This is not a disease that affects "us" and "them." We are them and they are us. AIDS is a human disease.

When history looks back to write the story of AIDS in this country and around the world, heroes will be recorded. There will also be thousands of unrecorded heroes. Nurses and other health care providers who on a daily basis deliver life-enhancing and life-giving care to PWAs in all settings are the real heroes in this epidemic. While many of you may never be commemorated by name and fame may never be yours, you will be recorded in our hearts and those of our family and friends.

REFERENCE

1. Levine, S. & Ram Dass (1986). Exploring the heart of healing. Novato, CA: The Access Group. *San Francisco Chronicle* (Nov. 14, 1990). AIDS steroid report was delayed by panel.

This chapter appears in Flaskerud, J.H. and Ungvarski, P.J. *HIV/AIDS: A guide to nursing care*. 2nd edition. Philadelphia: W.B. Saunders, 1992, pp 440–457. Reprinted with permission.

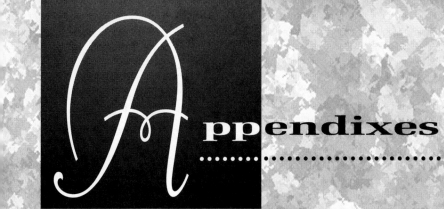

Appendixes

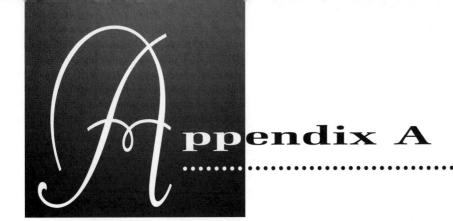

Appendix A

Journal Publishers

Current Science
20 North Third St.
Philadelphia, PA 19106-2199
Phone: (800) 552-5866

Publishes the journal *AIDS*.

Medical Publishing Group
1440 Main St.
Waltham, MA 02154-1649
Phone: (617) 893-3800

A division of the Massachusetts
Medical Society, this company
publishes *AIDS Clinical Care*, reprints
*Morbidity and Mortality Weekly
Report*, publishes several
AIDS-related books, and has two
compact disk and computer
communications products, the
*Compact Library: AIDS and AIDS
Knowledge Base*. Among its books is
The AIDS Knowledge Base (Cohen,
Sande, & Volberding, 1990).

Raven Press
1185 Avenue of the Americas
New York, NY 10036
Phone: (212) 930-9500

Publishes the *Journal of Acquired
Immune Deficiency Syndromes*.

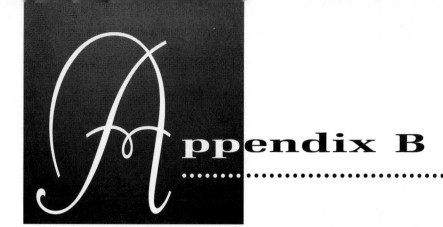

Appendix B

Newsletter Publishers

American Health Consultants, Inc.
60 Peachtree Park Dr. NE
Atlanta, GA 30309-1397
Phone: (404) 926–1775

Publishes *AIDS Alert* and *AIDS Medical Report.*

CDC AIDS Weekly Subscription
  Office
P.O. Box 830409
Charles Henderson Publications
P.O. Box 830409
Birmingham, AL 35283-0409
Phone: (800) 633-4931/
        (205) 991-6920

Publishes the weekly newsletter *AIDS Weekly*.

National Association of People with
  AIDS (NAPWA)
1413 K Street NW, 8th floor
Washington, DC 20005-3405
Phone: (202) 898-0414

Williams & Wilkins
P.O. Box 23291
428 E. Preston St.
Baltimore MD 21202
Phone: (410) 528–4000

Publishes *ATTN: AIDS Targeted Information Newsletter*, which contains literature reviews.

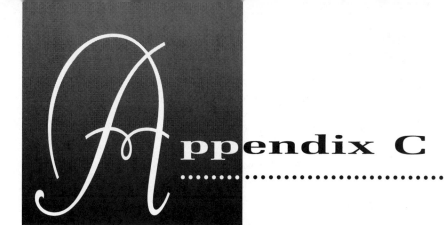

ppendix C

Helping Organizations

American Foundation for AIDS Research
733 Third Avenue, 12th floor
New York, NY 10017
Phone: (212) 682-7440

Funds research projects and publishes several compendiums of information, including AIDS information resource and experimental treatment directories. Also sponsors *ATTN: AIDS Targeted Information Newsletter*, a compendium of abstracts and citations, and *AIDS Clinical Care*, a newsletter.

American Social Health Association
P.O. Box 13827
Research Triangle Park, NC 27709
Phone: (919) 361-8400

ASHA publishes pamphlets and other information regarding sexually transmitted diseases, including AIDS, herpes, and genital warts.

Body Positive
P.O. Box 493
London, England W14 OTH UK
Phone: 01-373 9124

A voluntary organization run by HIV-positive persons, with a telephone help-line open evenings.

Canadian AIDS Society
100 Spark St., Suite 701
Ottawa, Canada K1P 5B7
Phone: (613) 230-3580

A coalition of community-based groups fighting AIDS. Lists member organizations throughout Canada and has publications.

Gay Men's Health Crisis (GMHC)
129 W. 20th St.
New York, NY 10011-0022
Phone: (212) 807-6655

One of the first groups to coalesce because of the epidemic. Wide range of quality publications available, as well as a hotline and social services. Published the booklet, *Medical Answers About AIDS*.

Names Project
310 Townsend St., Suite 310
San Francisco, CA 94107
Phone: (415) 882–5500

The Names Project is responsible for the AIDS Quilt, which memorializes those who died of AIDS.

National Association of People with AIDS (NAPWA)
1413 K Street NW, 8th floor
Washington, DC 20005-3405
Phone: (202) 898-0414

National Council on Death and Dying
200 Varick St.
New York, NY 10014
Phone: (212) 366-5540

Provides educational materials, a newsletter, living will forms, and a living will registry.

People with AIDS Coalition
31 West 26th St., Fifth floor
New York, NY 10010
Phone: (212) 532-0290

Project Inform
347 Dolores St., Suite 301
San Francisco, CA 94110
Phones: National: (800) 822-7422
California: (800) 334-7422
San Francisco: (415) 558-9051

San Francisco AIDS Foundation
25 Van Ness Ave., Suite 660
P.O. Box 426182
San Francisco, CA 94142-6182
Phone: (415) 861-3397

Its *AIDS Educator* catalog includes more than 65 education and training tools, with emphasis on cultural sensitivity and nonhomophobic language.

Terrence Higgins Trust Ltd.
52-54 Grays Inn Road
London, England WC1N 8JU
Phone: 01-242 1010

A charity that provides information and advice. Has a series of booklets and a helpline.

UCSF AIDS Health Project
Box 0884
San Francisco, CA 94143-0884
Phone: (415) 476-6430

Publishes a newsletter entitled *Focus*, as well as books, video/audio cassettes, and brochures.

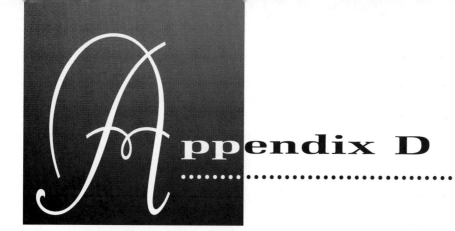

Appendix D

Political Action Groups

ACT UP
135 West 29th St.
New York, NY 10001
Phone: (212) 564-2437

Provides information and specializes in confrontative actions.

People with AIDS Coalition
31 West 26th St., Fifth floor
New York, NY 10010
Phone: (212) 532-0290

An organization of HIV-positive persons and others that provide information and assistance.

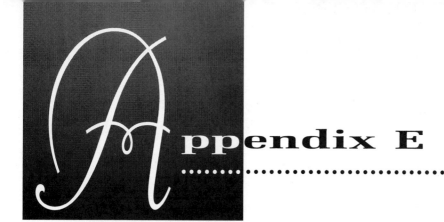

Appendix E

Professional Organizations

American Nurses Association HIV Task Force
600 Maryland Avenue SW,
Suite 100 West
Washington, DC 20024-2571
Phone: (800) 274-4262

American Psychiatric Association AIDS Steering Committee
1400 K St. NW
Washington, DC 20005
Phone: (202) 682-6143

APA has published *A Psychiatrist's Guide to AIDS and HIV Disease*, a training program, a computerized self-help test on the psychiatric aspects of AIDS, and training videos.

American Psychological Association
750 First St. NE
Washington, DC 20002
Phone: (202) 336-6057

The Association has an office specifically for AIDS, which has a computerized AIDS Resource Network listing

those who work with HIV disease, and a publication entitled *Psychology & AIDS Exchange*. Also, APA publishes PsycINFO, a psychological abstracts information service, and the book *AIDS: Abstracts of the Psychological and Behavioral Literature* with updates.

Association of Nurses in AIDS Care
704 Stony Hill Road, Suite 106
Yardley, PA 19067
Phone: (215) 321-2371

Has annual meetings, local chapters, and publishes a journal.

New York State Psychological Association Task Force on AIDS
Barbara Eisold, Ph.D
285 Central Park West
New York, NY 10024

(See also American Psychological Association)

**Physicians Association for AIDS
  Care**
101 West Grand Ave., Suite 200
Chicago, IL 60610
Phone: (312) 222-1326

Organization of physicians that
provides AIDS-related programming
via broadcast and print media to
members.

Site	Service Area
Pennsylvania/New York ETC **AIDS Training Center A-158** **Albany Medical Center** **47 New Scotland Avenue** **Albany, NY 12208** **Phone: (518) 445-4675**	Albany, NY area
University of Pittsburgh AIDS ETC **Graduate School of Public Health** **130 De Soto Street** **Pittsburgh, PA 15260** **Phone: (412) 624-1895**	Pennsylvania, upstate New York
Western AIDS ETC **University of California – Davis** **California Area Health Ed. System** **5110 East Clinton Way, Suite 115** **Fresno, CA 93727-2098** **Phone: (209) 252-2851**	California (excluding 5 southern counties), Nevada, Arizona, Hawaii
New York-Caribe AIDS/SIDA ETC **429 Shimkin Hall, Washington Square** **New York University** **New York, NY 10003** **Phone: (212) 998-5335**	New York City, Long Island, New Jersey, Puerto Rico, Virgin Islands
UW AIDS ETC **1001 Broadway** **Seattle, WA 98104** **Phone: (206) 543-9750**	Washington, Alaska, Montana, Idaho, Oregon

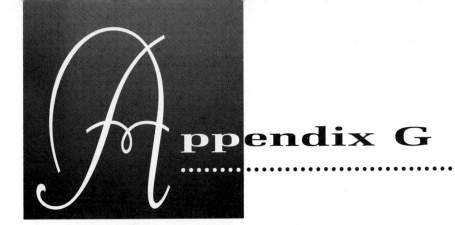

Appendix G

Special Interest Groups

**Association for Drug Abuse
  Prevention and Treatment**
552 Southern Blvd.
Bronx, NY 10455
Phone: (718) 665–5421

National Hemophilia Foundation
110 Greene Street, Room 406
New York, NY 10012
Phone: (212) 966-9247

Provides informational publications
regarding hemophilia and HIV. Will
direct you to local chapters and
regional comprehensive care centers
for the person with hemophilia.
Operates the hemophilia and AIDS/
HIV Network for the Dissemination
of Information, which offers
publications, bibliographies, article
reprints, and other resources.

Minority Task Force on AIDS
505 Eighth Ave., 16th floor
New York, NY 10018
Phone: (212) 563-8340

Women and AIDS Resource Network
P.O. Box 020525
Brooklyn, NY 11202
30 Third Ave., Suite 212
Brooklyn, NY 11217
Phone: (718) 596-6007

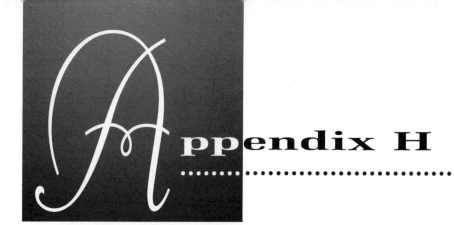

Appendix H

Substance Abuse Publications

Manisses Communications Group, Inc.
205 Governor St.
P.O. Box 3357
Providence, RI 02906-0357

Publishes *The Brown University Digest of Addiction Theory and Application*, a digest of addiction research found in more than 75 journals.

Substance Abuse Services
Department of Psychiatry
San Francisco General Hospital
1001 Potrero Ave.
San Francisco, CA 94110
Phone: (415) 206-3157

Has a catalog of some 75 publications dealing with substance abuse available for the price of photocopying. Also included are books and unpublished manuscripts.

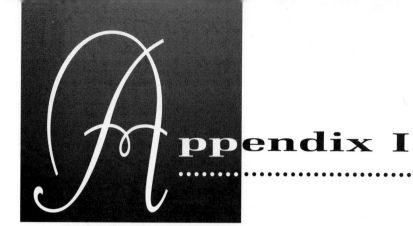

$\mathscr{A}$ppendix I

Technical Information

Agency for Health Care Policy and Research
Publications and Information Branch
18–12 Parklawn Building
Rockville, MD 20857
Phone: (301) 443-4100

This branch of the U.S. Public Health Service funds research on problems related to quality, delivery, and costs of health services. It publishes *Research Activities*, a monthly newsletter, and notices of special research interests.

National AIDS Information Clearinghouse
U.S. Department of Health and Human Services
Public Health Service, Centers for Disease Control
P.O. Box 6003
Rockville, MD 20849-6003
Phone: (800) 458-5231
Fax: (301) 738-6616

TTY/TTD: (800) 243-7012
International Line: (301) 217-0023

Identifies organizations doing AIDS-related works, locates educational materials, offers citations and descriptions of resources for education of children, describes U.S. funding opportunities, and publishes information publications such as a conference calendar.

National Library of Medicine
8600 Rockville Pike
Bethesda, MD 20894
Phone: (301) 496-6308

With a legislative mandate to create an AIDS-related base, the library provides several online computer files, dealing with AIDS literature, information on clinical trials of drugs and vaccines, and resource organizations. It also produces a monthly bibliography and publishes a listing of health hotlines.

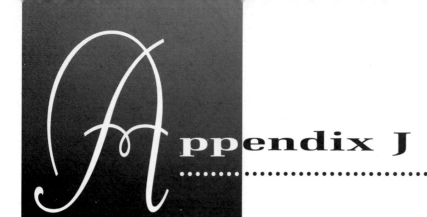

Appendix J

Telephone Information Lines

American Social Health Association
   National Sexually Transmitted
   Diseases Hotline: (800) 227–8922

Cocaine Hotline: (800) COCAINE

National Information Service for:
   National Library of Medicine, the
   Food and Drug Administration,
   and the Centers for Disease
   Control.
HIV-positive persons can obtain
information about availability of
clinical trials of medications: (800)
TRIALS-A.

Gay Men's Health Crisis Hotline
New York, NY
Phone: (212) 807-6655

National AIDS Hotline, service of
   the U.S. Public Health Service
   Centers for Disease Control:
(800) 342-AIDS;
in Spanish: (800) 344-SIDA.

National Native American AIDS
   Prevention Center
Indian AIDS Hotline:
   (800) 283-AIDS

Pediatric AIDS Hotline:
(718) 430-3333

People With AIDS Coalition Hotline:
(800) 828-3280

Project Inform Information Hotline
National: (800) 822-7422
California: (800) 334-7422
San Francisco: (415) 558-9051

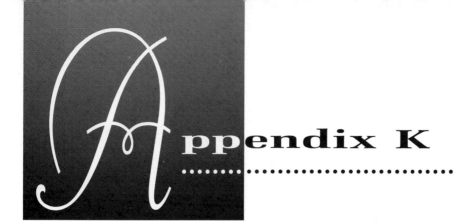

Appendix K

Women's Issues

Association for Women's AIDS
   Research and Education
3180 18th St., Suite 205
San Francisco, CA 94110
Phone: (415) 476-4091

Haitian Women's Program
465 Dean St.
Brooklyn, NY 11217
Phone: (718) 783–0883

National Research Center on
   Women and AIDS
2000 P Street NW, Suite 508
Washington, DC 20036
Phone: (202) 872-1770

Women and AIDS Resource Network
P.O. Box 020525
30 Third Ave., Suite 212
Brooklyn, NY 11217
Phone: (718) 596-6007

Women's AIDS Network
San Francisco AIDS Foundation
P.O. Box 426182
San Francisco, CA 94142-6182
Phone: (415) 864-4376, Ext. 2007

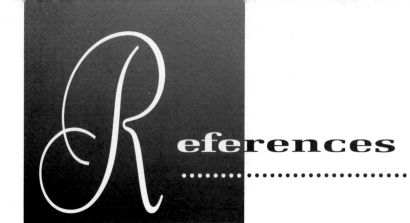

eferences

American Nurses Association. *Nursing and the human immunodeficiency virus: A guide for nursing's response to AIDS*. Washington, DC: American Nurses Association, 1988.

Beckett, A., & Rutan, J.S. (1990) Treating people with ARC and AIDS in group psychotherapy. *International Journal of Group Psychotherapy*, 1990, *40*, 19–28.

Callahan, M., & Kelley, P. *Final gifts: Understanding the special awareness, needs, and communications of the dying*. New York: Poseidon Press, 1992.

Child, R., & Getzel, G.S. Group work with inner city persons with AIDS. *Social Work with Groups*, 1990, *12*, 65–80.

Donovan, M.I., & Pierce, S.G. *Cancer care nursing*. New York: Appleton Century Crofts, 1984.

Douglas, C.J., Kalman, C.M., & Kalman, T. Homophobia among physicians and nurses: An empirical study. *Hospital and Community Psychiatry*, 1985, *36*, 1309–11.

Erickson, E.H. *Young man Luther: A study in psychoanalysis and history*. New York: W.W. Norton, 1958.

Flaskerud, J.H. Psychosocial aspects. In Flaskerud, J.H., & Ungvarski, P.J. (Eds.). *HIV/AIDS: A guide to nursing care*. Philadelphia: W.B. Saunders, 1992.

Gambe, R., & Getzel, G.S. Group work with gay men with AIDS. *Social Casework*, 1989, *70*, 172–179.

Gavzer, B. What keeps me alive. *Parade*. Jan. 31, 1993, 4–7.

Hays, R. Behaviors perceived as helpful and non-helpful to HIV-infected persons by friends and families. *A Message to the HIV Frontline* #11, Jan/Feb, 1993.

Kendall, J., Gloersen, B., Gray, P., McConnell, S., Turner, J., & West, J. Doing well with AIDS: Three case illustrations. *Archives of Psychiatric Nursing*, 1989, *3*(3), 159–165.

Kübler-Ross, E. *AIDS: The ultimate challenge*. New York: Macmillan, 1987.

Lego, S. Group psychotherapy with HIV-infected persons and their care-givers. In *Comprehensive group psychotherapy* (3rd ed.). Kaplan, H., & Sadock, B. (Eds.). Baltimore: Williams & Wilkens, 1993.

Lego, S. Group therapy. In *The American handbook of psychiatric nursing*. Lego, S. (Ed.). Philadelphia: J.B. Lippincott, 1984.

Mavia, B.A., Jordan, B.D., & Price, R.W. AIDS dementia complex: I Clinical features. *Annuals of Neurology*, 1986, *19*, 517–524.

Nichols, S.E. Psychiatric aspects of AIDS. *Psychosomatics*, 1983, *24*, 1083–1089.

Posey, E.C. Confidentiality in an AIDS support group. *Journal of Counseling and Development*, 1988, *66*, 226–227.

Rosenberg, P.R. Support groups: A special therapeutic entity. *Small Group Behavior*, 1984, *15*, 173–186.

Sontag, S. *Illness as metaphor and AIDS and its metaphors*. New York: Doubleday/Anchor Books, 1989.

Spector, I.C., & Conklin, R. Brief reports: AIDS group psychotherapy. *International Journal of Group Psychotherapy*, 1987, *37*(3), 433–439.

Tasker, M. *How can I tell you? Secrecy and disclosure with children when a family member has AIDS*. Bethesda, MD: Association for the Care of Children's Health, 1992.

Trice, A.D. Post-traumatic stress syndrome-like symptoms among AIDS care-givers. *Psychological Reports*, 1988, *63*, 656–658.

Tunnell, G. Complications in group psychotherapy with AIDS patients. *International Journal of Group Psychotherapy*, 1991, *41*, 481–497.

Winiarski, M.G. *AIDS-related psychotherapy*. New York: Pergamon Press, 1991.

Yalom, I. *The theory and practice of group psychotherapy*. New York: Basic Books, 1985.

CHILDREN'S BOOKS

Aliki. *The two of them*. New York: William Morrow, 1987.

Baker, L.S. *You and HIV: A day at a time*. Philadelphia: W.B. Saunders, 1991.

Buscalglia, L. *The fall of Freddie the Leaf*. New York: Henry Holt, 1982.

Clifton, L. *Everett Anderson's goodbye*. New York: Henry Holt.

Hausherr, R. *Children and the AIDS virus*. New York: Houghton Mifflin, 1989.

Hazen, B.S. *Why did Grandpa die?* New York: Golden Books, 1985.

Krementz, J. *How it feels to fight for your life*. Boston: Little Brown, 1989.

LeSham, E. *When a parent is very sick*. Boston: Little Brown, 1986. (For adolescents.)

LeShan, E. *Learning to say goodbye*. New York: Macmillan, 1976. (For adolescents.)

Mayer, M. *There's a nightmare in my closet*. New York: Dial Books, 1968.

Merrifield, M. *Come sit by me*. Toronto: Women's Press, 1990.

Quackenbush, M., & Villareal, S. *Does AIDS hurt?* Santa Cruz, CA: Network Publications, 1988.

Rockwell, H. *My doctor*. New York: Harper & Row, 1973.

Rogers, F. *Going to the doctor's*. New York: G.P. Putnam, 1986.

Sims, A.M. *Am I still a sister?* Albuquerque: Big A & Co., 1986.

Stein, S.B. *About dying*. New York: Walker, 1974.

Tasker, M. *Jimmy and his family*. Available from the Association for the Care of Children's Health, 7910 Woodmont Avenue, Suite 300, Bethesda, MD 20814, (301) 654-6549.

Tasker, M. *Jimmy and the eggs virus*, 1988. Available from Children's Hospital AIDS Program, Children's Hospital of New Jersey, United Hospital Medical Center, 15 South 9th Street, Newark, NJ 07107, (201) 268–8273.

Viorst, J. *The tenth good thing about Barney*. New York: Macmillan, 1971.

Wilhelm, H. *I'll always love you*. New York: Crown Publishers, 1988.

Novels, Poetry, Plays, Movies, and Diaries about AIDS

Novels and Poetry

Hoffman, A. *At risk*. New York: Bantam Books, 1988.

Klein, M. *Poets for life: Seventy-six poets respond to AIDS*. New York: Crown Publishers, 1989.

Monette, P. *Afterlife*. New York: Crown Publishers, 1990.

Plays

Kramer, L. *The Normal Heart*.

Kramer, L. *The Destiny of Me*.

Movies

Longtime Companion.

An Early Frost.

Andre's Mother.

Diaries and Memoirs, Personal Accounts

Brown, J. (Ed.) A promise to remember: The Names Project Book of Letters. New York: Avon, 1992.

Callen, M. (Ed.). *Surviving and thriving with AIDS: Hints for the newly diagnosed*. New York: People with AIDS Coalition, 1987.

Cox, E. *Thanksgiving: An AIDS journal*. New York: Harper & Row, 1990.

Dreuilhe, E. *Mortal embrace: Living with AIDS*. New York: Hill & Wang, 1988.

Holleran, A. *Ground zero: Essays*. New York: William Morrow, 1988.

Landau, E. *We had AIDS*. New York: Franklin Watts, 1990.

McCarroll, T. *Morning glory babies: Children with AIDS and the celebration of life*. New York: St. Martin's Press, 1988.

Monette, P. *Borrowed time: An AIDS memoir*. New York: Harcourt Brace Jovanovich, 1988.

Oyler, C. *Go toward the light*. New York: Harper & Row, 1988.

Peabody, B. *The screaming room: A mother's journal of her son's struggle with AIDS: A true story of love, dedication and courage*. San Diego: Oak Tree Publishers, 1986.

Peavey, F. *A shallow pool of time*. San Francisco: Crabgrass Press, 1989.

Nungesser, L.G. *Epidemic of courage: Facing AIDS in America*. New York: St. Martin's Press, 1986.

Reed, P. *Serenity: Challenging the fear of AIDS—From despair to hope*. Berkeley, CA: Celestial Arts, 1987.

Reed, P. *The Q Journal: A treatment diary*. Berkeley, CA: Celestial Arts, 1991.

Shilts, R. *And the band played on: Politics, people and the AIDS epidemic*. New York: St. Martin's Press, 1987.

Tilleraas, P. *Circle of hope: Our stories of AIDS, addiction and recovery*. Center City, MN: Hazelden, 1990.

White, E. *The darker proof: Stories from a crisis*. New York: New American Library, 1988.

Whitmore, G. *Someone was here: Profiles in the AIDS epidemic*. New York: New American Books, 1988.

SUGGESTED READINGS FROM PROFESSIONAL LITERATURE

Allers, C.T. AIDS and the older adult. *Gerontologist*, 1990, *30*, 405–407.

Allport, G.W. *The nature of prejudice*. New York, Doubleday/Anchor Books, 1958.

American Psychiatric Association. AIDS policy: Confidentiality and disclosure. *American Journal of Psychiatry*, 1988, *145*, 54.

Batki, S.L., Sorensen, J.L., Faltz, B., & Madover, S. Psychiatric aspects of treatment of IV drug abusers with AIDS. *Hospital and Community Psychiatry*, 1988, *39*, 439–441.

Boland, M., Tasker, M., Evans, P., & Keresztes, J. Helping children with AIDS: The role of the child welfare worker. *Public Welfare*, 1987, *23*, 23–29.

Bor, R., Miller, R., & Goldman, E. *Theory and practice of HIV counselling*. New York, Brunner-Mazel, 1992.

Calabrese, J.R., Kling, M.A., & Gold, P.W. Alterations in immunocompetence during stress, bereavement, and depression: Focus on neuroendocrine regulation. *American Journal of Psychiatry*, 1987, *144*, 1123.

Dane, B.O. New beginnings for AIDS patients. *Social Casework*, 1989, *70*, 305–309.

DeSpelcler, L.A., & Strickland, A.L. *The last dance: Encountering death and dying* (2nd ed.). Mountain View, CA: Mayfield Publishing, 1983.

Detwiler, D.A. The positive function of denial. *Journal of Pediatrics*, 1981, *99*, 401–402.

Douard, J.W. AIDS, stigma, and privacy. *AIDS and Public Policy Journal*, 1990, *5*(1), 37–41.

Dunkel, J., & Hatfield, S. Countertransference issues in working with persons with AIDS. *Social Work*, 1986, *31*, 114–116.

Durham, J.D., & Cohen, F.L. *The person with AIDS: Nursing perspectives*. New York: Springer Verlag, 1987.

Edison, T. (Ed.). *The AIDS care-giver's handbook*. New York: St. Martin's Press, 1988.

Farrell, B. AIDS patients: Values in conflict. *Critical Care Nursing Quarterly*, 1987, *10*, 74–85.

Feinblum, S. Pinning down the psychosocial dimensions of AIDS. *Nursing and Health Care*, 1988, *7*, 225.

Ferrara, A. My personal experience with AIDS. *American Psychologist*, 1984, *39*(11), 1285–1287.

Forstein, M. The psychological impact of the acquired immunodeficiency syndrome. *Seminars in Sociology*, 1984, *11*(1), 77–82.

Frierson, R., & Lippman, S. Psychological implications of AIDS. *American Family Practitioner*, 1987, *35*(3), 109–116.

Frierson, R.L., Lippman, S.B., & Johnson, J. Psychological stresses on the family. *Psychosomatics*, 1987, *28*, 65–68.

Gaffney, D. *The seasons of grief: Helping children grow through loss*. New York: New American Library, 1988.

Geis, S.B., Fuller, R.L., & Rush, J. Lovers of AIDS victims: Psychosocial stresses and counseling needs. *Death Studies*, 1986, *10*, 43–53.

Goffman, E. *Stigma*. Englewood Cliffs, NJ: Prentice-Hall, 1963.

Gonda, T.A., & Ruark, J.E. *Dying dignified. The health professional's guide to care*. Menlo Park: Addison-Wesley, 1984.

Grant, D. Support group for youth with AIDS virus. *International Journal of Group Psychotherapy*, 1988, *38*, 237–251.

Hagglund, T. *Dying: A psychoanalytical study with special reference to individual creativity and defensive organization*. New York: International Universities Press, 1978.

Haney, P. Providing empowerment to the person with AIDS. *Social Work*, 1988, *33*, 251–253.

Jackson, E.N. *Telling a child about death*. New York: Channel Press, 1965.

Keith-Lucas, A. *Giving and taking help*. Chapel Hill, NC: University of North Carolina Press, 1972.

Kelber, M.B., & McIntyre, R. Point/counterpoint: Nurse-assisted suicide. *Journal of the Association of Nurses in AIDS Care*, 1992, *3* (1), 23–24.

Kellerman, J., Rigler, D., Siegel, S.E., & Katz, E.R. Disease-related communication and depression in pediatric cancer patients. *Journal of Pediatric Psychology*, 1977, *2* (2), 52–53.

Kelly, J.A., St. Lawrence, J.S., Smith, S., Hood, H.V., & Cook, D.J. Stigmatization of AIDS patients by physicians. *American Journal of Public Health*, 1987, *77*, 789.

Kennedy, M. AIDS: Coping with the fear. *Nursing 87* 1987, April, 45–46.

Knox, M.D. Community mental health's role in the AIDS crisis. *Community Mental Health Journal*, 1989, *25*, 185.

Kristal, A. The impact of acquired immunodeficiency syndrome on patterns of premature death in New York City. *Journal of the American Medical Association*, 1986, *255* (17), 2306–2310.

Kübler-Ross, E. *On death and dying*. New York: Macmillan, 1969.

Landau-Stanton, J., & Clements, C.D. *AIDS Health and Mental Health*. New York: Brunner-Mazel, 1993.

Lauritsen, J. Poison by prescription: The AZT story. New York: Asklepios, 1990.

McFarland, R. *Coping with stigma*. New York: The Rosen Publishing Group, 1989.

Magura, S., Shapiro, J.L., Grossman, J.I., & Lipton, D.S. Education/support groups for AIDS prevention with at-risk clients. *Social Casework*, 1989, *70*, 10–20.

Maj, M. Psychological problems of families and health workers dealing with people infected with human immunodeficiency virus. *Acta Psychiatric Scandanavia*, 1991, *83*, 161–167.

Mantrell, J.E., Schulman, L.C., Belmont, M.F., & Spivak, H.B. Social workers respond to the AIDS epidemic in an acute care hospital. *Health and Social Work*, 1989, *14*, 41–51.

Marzuk, P.M., Tierney, H., Tardiff, K., Gross, E., Morgan, E., Hsu, M.A., & Mann, J. Increased risk of suicide in persons with AIDS. *Journal of the American Medical Association*, 1988, *259* (9), 1333–1337.

Molnos, A. *Our response to a deadly virus: The group-analytic approach*. London: Karnac Books, 1990.

Morin, S., Charles, K., & Malyon, A. The psychological impact of AIDS on gay men. *American Psychologist*, 1984, *39*(11), 1289–1293.

Nichols, S. Psychiatric aspects of AIDS. *Psychosomatics*, 1983, *24*, 1083–1089.

Nichols, S. Psychosocial reactions of persons with acquired immunodeficiency syndrome. *Annals of Internal Medicine*, 1985, *103*(5), 765–767.

O'Dowd, M. Psychosocial issues in HIV-infection. *AIDS 1988*, 1988, *2*(Suppl 1), 201–205.

Pearlin, L.I., Semple, S., & Tumer, H. Stress of AIDS caregiving: A preliminary overview of the issues. *Death Studies*, 1988, *12*, 501–517.

Pearson, J.M. *Talking to terminally ill children about death*. Paper presented at the meeting of the American Academy of Child Psychiatry, Dallas, 1981.

Perry, S.W., & Markowitz, J. Psychiatric interventions for AIDS-spectrum disorders. *Hospital and Community Psychiatry*, 1986, *37*, 1001.

Price, R.E., Omizo, M.M., & Hammett, V.L. Counseling clients with AIDS. *Journal of Counseling and Development*, 1986, *65*, 96–97.

Riley, M., Ory, M., & Zublotsky, D. (Eds.). *AIDS in an aging society: What we need to know*. New York: Springer Verlag, 1989.

Roback, H.B., Ochoa, E., Bloch, F., & Purdon, S. Guarding confidentiality in clinical groups: The therapist's dilemma. *International Journal of Group Psychotherapy*, 1992, *42*, 81–103.

Siegel, K. AIDS: The social dimension. *Psychiatric Annals*, 1986, *16*(3), 168–172.

Siegel, K. Rational suicide: Considerations for the clinician. *Psychiatric Quarterly*, 1982, *54*(2), 77–84.

Simmons-Alling, S. AIDS: Psychosocial needs of the health care worker. *Topics in Clinical Nursing*, 1984, *7*, 31.

Spinetta, J., & Deasy-Spinetta, P. *Emotional aspects of life-threatening illness in children*. Rockville, MD: Cystic Fibrosis Foundation, 1980.

Trieber, F.A., Shaw, D., & Malcolm, R. Acquired immune deficiency syndrome: Psychological impact on health personnel. *Journal of Nervous and Mental Disease*, 1987, *175*, 496.

Van Servellen, G., Lewis, C., & Leake, C. The stresses of hospitalization among AIDS patients on integrated and special care units. *International Journal of Nursing Studies*, 1990, *27*(3), 235–247.

Waechter, E.H. Children's awareness of fatal illness. *American Journal of Nursing*, 1971, *71*, 1168–1172.

Wong, M., & Forrister, D.K. Empowerment as a group work technique with persons with acquired immune deficiency syndrome. *Free Inquire in Creative Sociology*, 1989, *17*, 193–199.

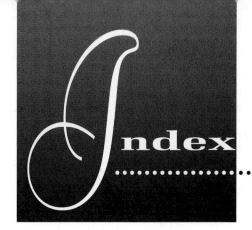

Index